SFIMMS SERIES IN NEUROMUSCULOSKELETAL MEDICINE

MYOFASCIAL AND FASCIAL-LIGAMENTOUS APPROACHES

IN OSTEOPATHIC

MANIPULATIVE MEDICINE

Harry D. Friedman, D.O.
Wolfgang G. Gilliar, D.O.
Jerel H. Glassman, D.O.

Published by SFIMMS Press

San Francisco International Manual Medicine Society

email: admin@sfimms.com
www.sfimms.com.

First Edition

Library of Congress Card Catalog Number 00-131503
ISBN 0-9701841-1-5

San Francisco International Manual Medicine Society

The San Francisco International Manual Medicine Society (SFIMMS) is an association of physicians and health professionals founded in 1995 to establish high educational standards and practice in the field of manual medicine.

The Society's courses are designed to provide health professionals with a strong foundation in manual medicine. The courses are offered at basic, intermediate and advanced levels with appropriate textbooks and course manuals provided. The educational format utilizes a variety of approaches including: Didactic Teaching, Step-By-Step Presentation, Hands-on Laboratory Sessions and Clinical Problem Solving.

These high quality educational programs facilitate the acquisition of palpatory skills and clinical problem solving approaches using a low student-teacher ratio in a direct, hands-on format.

Founding Members

Wolfgang G. Gilliar, DO (right)

Dr. Gilliar is in private practice in San Mateo, CA. He is board certified in Physical Medicine and Rehabilitation, and Osteopathic Manipulative Medicine. He is an assistant clinical professor at Michigan State University College of Osteopathic Medicine. He is also the editor and co-author of many Manual Medicine texts and scientific papers. Dr. Gilliar lectures and teaches extensively at national and international meetings. His specific research interests include neurophysiologic processes in their application to manual medicine and exercise principles, as well as practice parameter development.

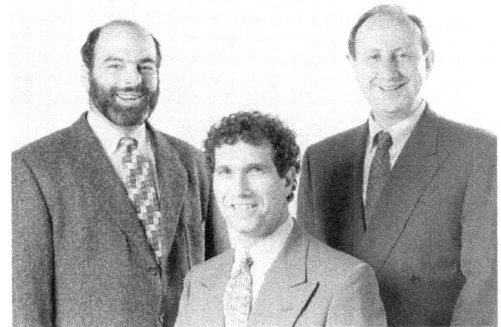

Harry D. Friedman, DO (left)

Dr Friedman is in private practice in Corte Madera, CA. He is board certified in Family Practice and Osteopathic Manipulative Medicine. He is an assistant clinical professor at Michigan State University College of Osteopathic Medicine and clinical faculty at Touro University College of Osteopathic Medicine.

Dr. Friedman has participated in various research studies concerning uniform osteopathic documentation. He is the author of a chapter for the <u>Foundations of Osteopathic Medicine</u> textbook and has co-authored the text <u>Functional Methods</u>. Dr. Friedman lectures and teaches extensively in the US and abroad, and is one of the faculty developing manual medicine programs for the American Academy of Family Physicians.

Jerel H. Glassman, MPH, DO (middle)

Dr. Glassman is a staff physician at St. Mary's Spine Center in San Francisco, CA. He is board certified in Physical Medicine and Rehabilitation, and Osteopathic Manipulative Medicine, and is an assistant clinical professor at Michigan State University College of Osteopathic Medicine and clinical faculty at Touro University College of Osteopathic Medicine. He is also a clinical instructor at Stanford University Medical School.

Dr. Glassman lectures frequently at many national meetings, including the American Academy of Physical Medicine and Rehabilitation, the American Back Society, the California Medical Association and American Osteopathic Association among others. Through his clinical and teaching activities he has pursued the integration of manual medicine into the multi-disciplinary rehabilitation model.

Foreward

The inspiration for this and the other books in the SFIMMS series in Neuromusculoskeletal Medicine came from our students and their desire for educational excellence. Quality instruction requires a level of clarity and correctness that reflects the subject's complexity but also allows for its comprehension on many different levels; conceptual, perceptual, and practical.

This material and the format in which it is presented have been developed to facilitate an understanding of Osteopathic Manipulative Medicine that encompasses its philosophy, science, and its practical clinical application. It is not the author's intention in writing this book to impart an Osteopathic education. Rather, we realize that such learning requires extensive study, supervision and clinical experience and cannot be acquired by simply reading this, or any other, book. We caution against the non-professional use of this book as it is intended as a textbook for Neuromusculoskeletal instruction in conjunction with a scientific education in the healing arts. Independent self-study of these
approaches without the proper background and supervision is expressly against the authors' recommendation and wishes.

We wish to acknowledge the support and inspiration of our teachers Robert Ward, DO FAAO and Anthony Chila, DO FAAO. They inspired us with their orginal contributions to the myofascial concept and enabled us to more fully appreciate the balancing beauty of the living system.

We have been enlightened by the writings of A.T. Still, William Garner Sutherland and Rollin Becker. And our palpatory experince has been expanded by Drs Frymann, Upledger, Jealous, Fulford, Barral, Greenman, Mitchell, Beal and Johnston among others. We are indebted to our teachers.

We wish to especially thank our wives, Denise, Barbara, and Beth for their support, and Eric Shilland for many hours of computer assistance

Contents

Level I

Level II

Contents

Objectives
Level I

Understand the anatomy and physiology
of myofascial and connective tissues
and their related neuroreflexive and
mechanical properties.

Understand the principles of the myofascial
release concept in osteopathic diagnosis and
treatment

Develop manipulative and problem
solving skills applying the myofascial
release concept to the spinal,
appendicular, costal and pelvic regions.

Appreciate the functional inter-relationships of
different body regions and the dynamic unity of
the whole body, in diagnosis and treatment.

Experience multiple operator procedures as both
an operator and as the subject.

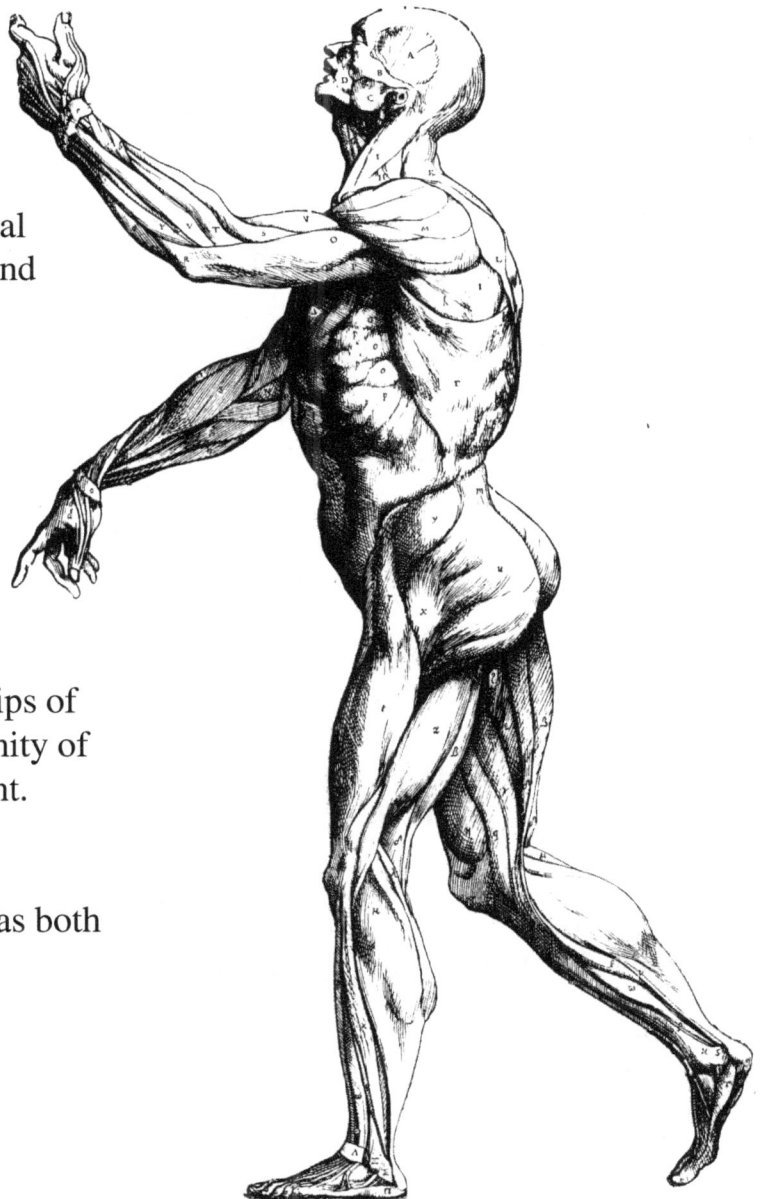

MYOFASCIAL RELEASE CONCEPT

Myofascial and Fascial Ligamentous Release is a manipulative approach which addresses the three-dimensional mobile function/dysfunction of both active (neuroreflexive, neuromuscular) and passive (viscoelastic, connective tissue) components of the musculoskeletal system.

Three-dimensional layering of myofascial tissue is assessed for relative balance (tightness and looseness) between left and right, front and back, as well as proximal and distal structures.

Treatment with Myofascial and Fascial Ligamentous Release uses direct stretching and pumping as well as indirect and direct unwinding techniques to effect neuroreflexive and viscoelastic changes underlying and distant from the point of contact. Three-dimensional perception of anatomic relationships is essential.

Treatment skills require assessment of superficial and deep myofascial tissues for functional balance, i.e., tightness and looseness, as well as sensing viscoelastic (i.e., creep, hysteresis) and neuroreflexive changes under sustained manual loads.

HISTORICAL CONTEXT

Myofascial relaxation and balancing techniques form the basis of the earliest described approaches to treatment using Osteopathic manual techniques. Barber (1898), one of the first graduates of A.T. Still's revolutionary medical program, describes these approaches to patient care in one of the first textbooks on Osteopathic techniques.

Throughout the twentieth century these approaches existed side by side with the better known ones applied to joint mobilization. In the later part of the century work by Sutherland, Becker, Ward and Chila further expanded this concept of neuroreflexive and neuromuscular responses.

These descriptions are meant as teaching instruments to assist students in their pursuit of the Osteopathic awareness of the body's great quest for balance.

A. <u>Neuroreflexive Properties</u>

Intrafusal muscle spindles lie parallel to the extrafusal muscle fibers (i.e. the contractile muscle) and increase afferent output as the extrafusal muscle is stretched. This allows the central nervous system to control the resistance to any given stretch by then contracting the extrafusal muscles. The intrafusal muscle spindle is capable of up- or downshifting its sensitivity to extrafusal muscle stretch (increasing or decreasing the "gain"), depending on the behavioral task anticipated by the nervous system. If a task requires maximal stretching of a muscle, then the gamma efferent mechanism, which controls intrafusal fiber muscle tone, will be set at a lower level of sensitivity in order to allow the muscle spindle to react less to stretching of the extrafusal fibers. On the other hand, if short quick bursts of muscle activity are needed without significantly stretching the muscle fiber, then the gamma efferent control will be set at a much higher sensitivity level in order to more quickly respond to small changes of muscle fiber stretching. Occasionally, in certain activities that are either unexpected or too quick for the spindle response to handle, the disparity between the resting length of the intrafusal and extrafusal muscle fibers can become too large, resulting in a permanent increase in sensitivity (gain) of the gamma control system. When this kind of disparity exists, the gamma efferent system becomes overly stimulated, and afferent discharge increases, causing extrafusal muscle contraction, which in turn brings the gamma system back towards its normal resting tone. Normal resting tone is never achieved this way, so continued gamma stimulation results in muscle spasm and related compensatory myofascial dysfunction. The inability of the gamma system to return to its normal resting tone is hypothesized as one mechanism for somatic dysfunction.

When we stretch the muscle in a controlled manner, as we do with Myofascial Release techniques, we automatically cause an increased output of the afferent intrafusal system connected to the gamma efferent control mechanism. If this stretch is sustained for a prolonged duration, the gamma motor neurons are unable to stimulate a reflex contraction in the extrafusal muscle fibers. Since the amount of stretch is below the threshold of the golgi tendon mechanism, the overloading and eventual fatigue of the gamma mechanism allows the resting tone (gain) to be reset at a lower level. Lengthening of the extrafusal matrix is accomplished by the Myofascial Release and the gamma system is able to correct the disparity that was previously influencing an overcontraction of the extrafusal fibers. Return of normal resting tone allows optimal synchronization between the intrafusal and extrafusal mechanisms and the surrounding myofascial tissues.

B. Properties of Connective Tissue: Definition of Terms

1. Stress: The internal forces interacting between contiguous parts of a body, caused by external forces, such as tension or shear. A force or system of forces causing strain.

2. Shear: A force causing two parts to slide on each other in opposite directions; the strain or deformation resulting from this shearing stress.

3. Strain: To cause alteration of form, shape or volume in a solid.

4. Stiffness: Stored (potential) energy within a tissue that creates a resistance to deformation; the load required to produce deformation.

5. Plastic: The capacity to be able to be deformed in any direction and to retain its deformed condition permanently.

6. Plastic deformation: The alteration of the shape of a solid by the application of a sufficient and sustained stress.

7. Viscoelastic: The mechanical response of a material, tissue, or structure which includes fluid resistance and restorative tendencies.

8. Relaxation: A decrease in resistive load over time with a constant deformation.

9. Linear stretch: Increase in length of a structure or tissue which is in the same direction as an applied force.

10. Creep: The slow continuous deformation of a tissue under stress below the yield point. The process of softening or flexing of material with accompanying change in shape that results from increased stress. Below a certain stress, creep will not take place at all.

11. Cyclic creep: Deformation that increases in response to a repeated load.

12. Hysteresis: A lagging of an effect behind its cause when a tissue is subjected to stress; energy is lost and the tissue is temporarily changed. (i.e., looser)

C. **Components of Connective Tissue**

Muscle resistance to stretch is only minimally due to neuroreflexive properties controlling muscle length. Resistance is more substantially influenced by the connective tissue framework than it is by the myofibrillar elements. In and around joints, connective tissues are the primary mobile restrictors which normally function to restrict as well as allow for motion. Forces of stress, tension and shear cause myofascial dysfunction (strain) which alters this mobile function through changes in connective tissue stiffness and viscoelasticity.

Connective tissue is made up of collagen fibers, elastin, and reticular fibers embedded in a protein-polysaccharide matrix, commonly referred to as "ground substance." Gel-Sol characteristics of ground substance allow it to act as both a fluid and a solid. Its function is optimized when its "sol" (fluid) state predominates. Collagen is a fibrous protein that has a very high tensile strength. Elastin and reticular fibers are also proteins but have a lower tensile strength with elastic properties that allow the tissue to return to its normal length after being stretched. When collagenous tissue is stretched, it behaves differently, and it undergoes permanent (plastic) deformation without returning completely to its previous configuration (creep). Energy is either stored or lost (hysteresis) and the tissue becomes stiffer or relaxed.

Cellular components of connective tissue include cells with metabolic, immune, and inflammatory function, including fibroblasts, macrophages and white blood cells. As part of the body's intercellular space, connective tissue is traversed by both nerves and blood vessels, which makes it a site for neuro-circulatory activity, particularly inflammation and the metabolic delivery of nutrients and removal of waste products. Connective tissues also have nociceptive nerve endings.

D. Mechanical Behavior of Connective Tissue

There are viscous, plastic, and elastic components of connective tissue. Viscous deformation is permanent, elastic deformation recovers. Permanent deformation occurs when connective tissue undergoes excessive loading or is loaded repetitively resulting in focal areas of stress and strain. Tissues stiffen and become tight or creep and become loose. Areas of tightness are clinically relevant and may respond to manual procedures which focus therapeutic forces to cause creep to occur. Stored energy in the tissues is released causing relaxation and reduced tissue stiffness (hysteresis). Relative looseness is introduced into connective tissues promoting tissue balance and restorative tendencies.

Symmetrical and assymetrical forces impact connective tissue constantly through the active and passive elements of motor behavior (sitting, standing, walking, running, bending, twisting, and resting). Active elements engage neuromuscular patterns of motion which tend to include both inhibited and overstimulated elements interacting together in the same muscle. These patterns create compensatory focal areas of tension, compression and tightness as well as distraction and looseness. Decompensation is reflected in decreasing motor function (range, quality, balance, coordination) with associated disability and pain.

Passive connective tissue elements can become a focus for tightness or looseness exerting a compressive (pulling) or distractive (pushing) force on local tissues. Compression pulls surrounding tissues into tightness while distraction allows excessive motion to occur into surrounding tissues. Tightness also has a tethering effect that limits motion away from the tight area while looseness weakens normal stabilizing functions encouraging motion towards tight areas. Both are associated with muscle fatigue, weakness and compromised reflexes resulting in weight bearing and coordination imbalances. Clinically, pain is often perceived in loose areas of excessive tissue motion, presumably due to nociceptor stimulation.

Tightness and looseness may arise from other than purely mechanical factors related to motor function. For example, thermal phenomena: heat loosens tissues while cooling tightens them, and neurochemical factors may be associated with central, peripheral, and autonomic effects on active and passive mobile elements. Endocrine and immune system regulation may also affect neurosensory processing as well as metabolic and fluid functions within connective tissues. Total behavior is a dynamic interactive process of some complexity.

E. Functional Anatomy of Connective Tissue

Superficial fascia is loose, fatty fibroelastic connective tissue. Pacinian corpuscles are located deep within this tissue compartment and are pressure receptors. The superficial fascia functions to control superficial blood flow and temperature regulation and acts as a venous pump to return fluids to the heart.

The **deep fascial compartment** has more of a supportive function to join, as well as separate, different anatomical structures, forming attachment points for various muscles as well as protecting various organs and neurocirculatory structures. The deep fascia is a dense structure with a tougher quality, more compact, which wraps around structures, with a strong layer of investing tissue. Deep fascia also has anchoring "feet" in the veins, which helps in decongesting fluids through muscle contraction.

The **subserous fascial layer** is a loose fibroelastic tissue, like the superficial fascia, and surrounds all organs. As organs develop, they move through this subserous fascia and remain in this fascia for their lifetime. Subserous fascia provides lubrication for all organ surfaces and surrounds all deep nervous and circulatory structures. The subserous and the deep fascia are actually continous with one another. The subserous fascia provides the outer lining for internal organs and their compartments, including the peritoneum, the pericardium, etc. In actuality, all abdominal organs are retroperitoneal, because in fact they lie within the subserous fascia, which is superficial to the peritoneum.

With age, the elastic components of connective tissues decrease, while the contractile or viscous properties persist throughout life. Therefore, with age the tissues have less ability to return to their normal configuration and undergo plastic deformation as gravity exerts more and more of an effect on the postural function (i.e. increased thoracic kyphosis).

There are four particular areas of postural fascia with which we are concerned clinically. The first is the lumbodorsal fascia, which is an attachment site for posterior muscle groups of the thoracolumbar spine, pelvis and lower extremity. Additionally, it assists in spinal motion and coordination of lower exremity and trunk muscles in their activities related to movement and posture. The second is the iliotibial band. The third is the gluteal fascia, and the fourth is the cervicothoracic fascia.

PATIENT ASSESSMENT

Optimal posture is expressed through structural and functional symmetry of static and dynamic activities. Proper co-ordination of all musculoskeletal elements requires proprioception, flexibility, segmental reflexes and muscle balance. Myofascial tension influences all these functions uniquely resulting in relative imbalance, stiffness, immobility and neurologic facilitation.

Standard musculoskeletal screening for altered structural motion and tissue should be carried out as an overall patient assessment (see pg. 98). Myofascial screening tests apply rotatory and translatory forces to assess relative tissue compliance. Testing procedures assess mobile responses at the initiation of motion and throughout the mobile range. Relative three-dimensional compliance is compared left to right observing the side that encounters resistance first.

Ten-Step Myofascial Screening Exam

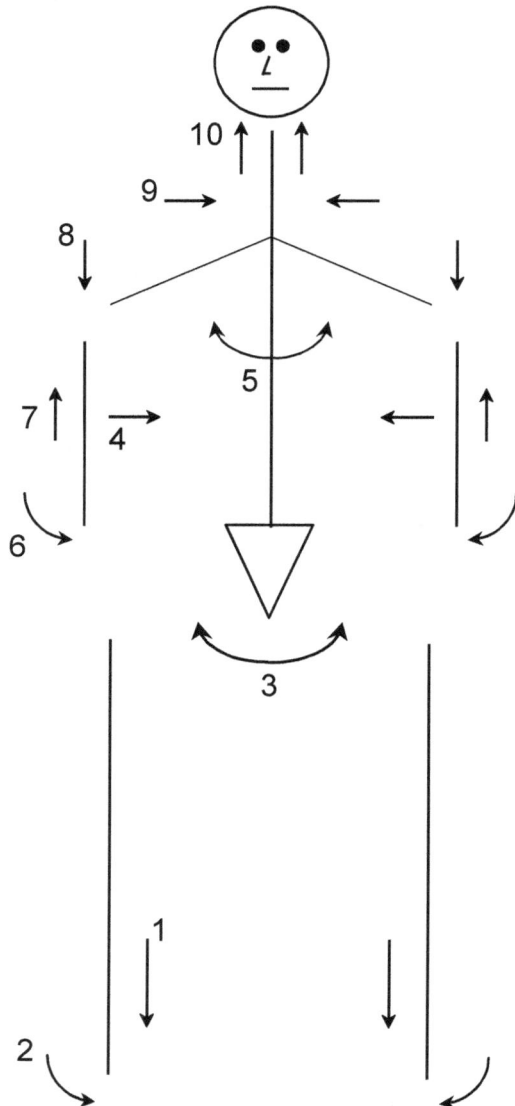

Compare findings for
↑ resistance (↓ compliance) L to R:

1. Traction test
2. Ankle inversion test
3. Pelvic rock
4. Costal cage translation
5. Costal cage compression
6. Forearm pronation
7. Shoulder abduction traction
8. Thoracic rock
9. Lateral cervical compression
10. Occipital traction

PRINCIPLES OF TREATMENT

A. The BBR Concept: Balance, Barrier, Release

1. All body tissues are in a state of balance at the beginning and end of any manual medicine procedure; however, they may be maladapative. Manual medicine procedures deliberately undo this balance in order to reach a more adaptive functional state.

2. Tissue barriers, any impediment to free biomechanical motion, are assessed during manual medicine procedures and are treated by either a direct or indirect approach. As a result, the barrier or tightness should be removed or its influence significantly reduced. (Throughout this manual, direct or indirect approaches are indicated for each table session, but each can be applied, interchangeably.)

3. At the conclusion of a myofascial or fascial ligamentous release procedure, barriers are released and a deeper sense of tissue balance and inherent motion results. These releases begin to occur at varying time intervals, averaging about 15 to 30 seconds, and are sensed as either a "melting away" of tissue tension or a release of myofascial tightness/ restrictions. Releases may be slow and deliberate or rapid and oscillating reflecting the tissues and body areas being treated. Initial force applied in any procedure is light and increased as tissue tension is engaged. Applied force is decreased if painful.

4. It is frequently true that a number of BBR sequences must occur before myofascial balance is achieved at a level that is associated with clinical functional improvement in the patient's chief complaint. This may also take repeated visits to accomplish.

B. Point of Entry with Tension, Traction, and Twist (POET3)

1. Contacting an area of maximum three-dimensional restriction constitutes a **point of entry** through which the treatment can begin with Myofascial and Fascial Ligamentous Release techniques. Midline or para-midline contact is important to stimulate the inherent healing and regulatory functions associated with the body's midline.

2. The use of **tension** to take up the slack in the tissues and then introducing **traction** (or compression) and **twist** in either a direct or indirect direction initiates the sequence of Myofascial and Fascial Ligamentous Release. Optimal localization of rotary and translatory forces allow the operator to appreciate tissue responses unique to each patient. Table height may be adjusted for best operator contact and least effort.

3. Techniques may use direct stretch along curvilinear planes of myofascial tension (this is where the twist comes in), or pumping techniques wherein the side that is "loose" is compressed to the barrier and the side that is "tight" is gently pumped with a slow compressive rhythmic force. Unwinding techniques use three-dimensional forces, coupling either direct or indirect forces to cause a sustained tissue release or unwinding. As unwinding begins, continue to apply compression (tension), letting go of the traction and twist. This unwinding should be followed until it comes to a point of rest, after which the tissues should be reassessed for three-dimensional symmetry. If asymmetry persists, the procedure should be repeated until tissue balance is improved.

PRINCIPLES OF TREATMENT

C. Proximal and Distal Releases

1. It is important that the operator remain focused and relaxed in order to enhance the ability to perceive and follow changes in the myofascial tissue. This requires a receptive mind and palpatory sense with which to follow inherent releases that are occuring underneath their hands. This is distinct fom "pushing tissues around" in the direction they should go or should be in. Any given Myofascial or Fascial Ligamentous Release may involve tissues at both a proximal and distal source, which makes release a unique and potentially far-reaching manual medicine procedure. Sensing tissue restrictions and releases along myofascial planes to distal regions of the body can be developed through visualizing total body anatomy and projecting palpatory awareness.

MYOFASCIAL TREATMENT OF THORAX AND COSTAL CAGE

1. Thoracolumbar Junction, Patient Prone Using a Direct Stretch Technique

Assessment of thoracolumbar mechanics is made by contacting the paraspinal tissues with the thenar eminences, thumbs pointing cephalward. From here, the rest of the hand falls laterally, contacting the rib cage at the mid-axillary line. Projecting palpatory awareness in this region, the operator should assess the overall sense of hardness/softness and tightness/looseness by gently rotating, side-bending, and compressing the tissues in the immediate area.

Treatment is achieved by placing a direct traction force between the two hands in a lateral and anterior direction through both the thenar eminences, as well as the pads of the hands and fingers, which extend anteriorly. There is an idea that the thoracic cage is a spherical object around which traction and twist is being applied and tissue is being stretched in a curvilinear manner. This traction should be maintained until there is a sense of inherent release under the hands, at which time the hands may move slightly in a superior/inferior or anterior/posterior manner through the process of inherent release. There may be a number of arcing releases, after which movement will cease and the region should be reassessed as before.

Oftentimes, there is a "red reflex" effect that occurs, particulary with this but also with other myofascial techniques. This is a redenning of the skin, which persists for longer that the typical vascular flaring that occurs after any pressure to the skin. This longer-lasting response is indicative of a neuroreflexive release that has occured in the tissues and may last for several minutes.

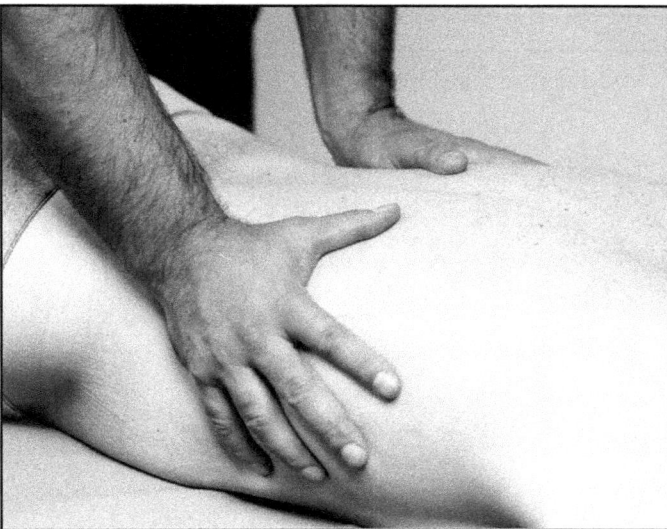

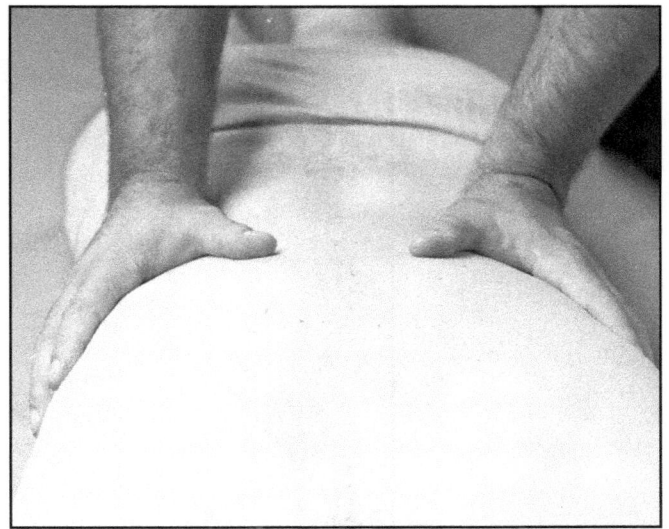

Prone Thoracolumbar Treatment

2. <u>Lower Costal Cage Release, Patient Supine Using an Indirect Technique</u>

The patient's anterior rib cage is **assessed** similarly to the last technique, with the thumbs pointing cephalward and the hands falling out laterally over the costal cage. Relative tensions and hardness of the tissues are assessed by testing relative degrees of compliance to various motions introduced, e.g. rotation, sidebending, traction, compression, lateral translation of the entire costal cage left and right, front to back.

Treatment is applied in an indirect manner, with directions of relative ease being combined and held and the inherent release followed until there is a return to balance and absence of mobile tissue release. The area should be reassessed after treatment.

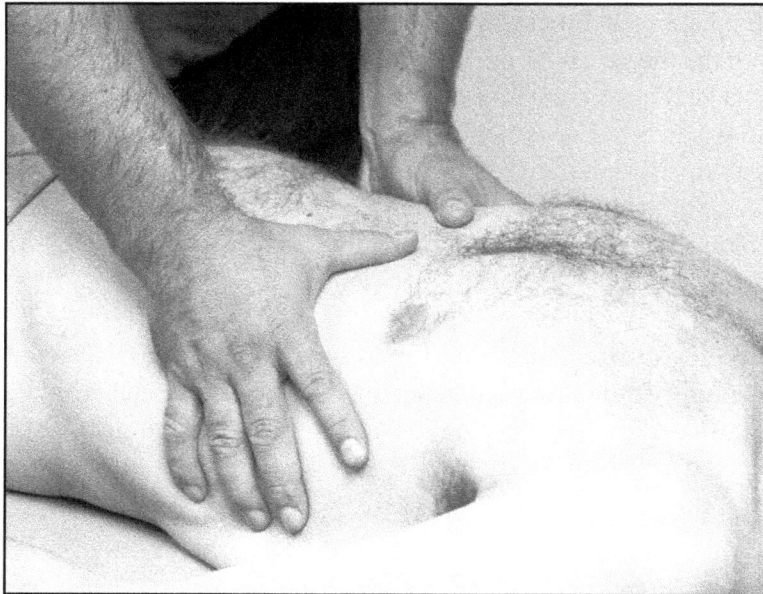

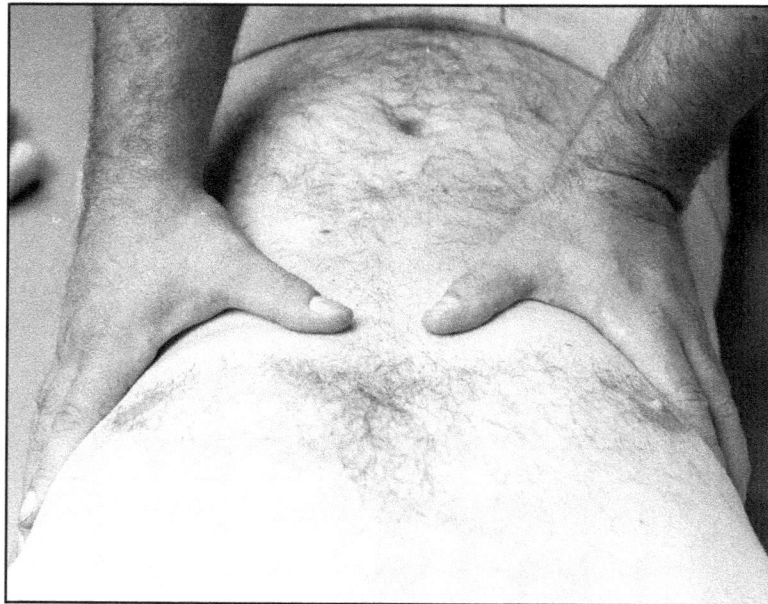

Supine Lower Costal Cage Treatment

3. Lower Costal Cage Treatment, Patient Seated Using an Indirect Technique

Operator stands behind the patient, reaching forward underneath the anterior lateral rib cage. **Assessment** of tissue compliance should be made by performing a simple translation test left and right, with treatment ensuing in the direction of ease.

For **treatment**, the patient should be instructed to exhale completely to begin the unwinding, allowing his head to fall forward. Unwinding may take the costal cage forward, backward, side-bending or rotating in various directions until the inherent release stops and is returned to a new point of balance. At this point the lateral translation test should be applied and assessed appropriately.

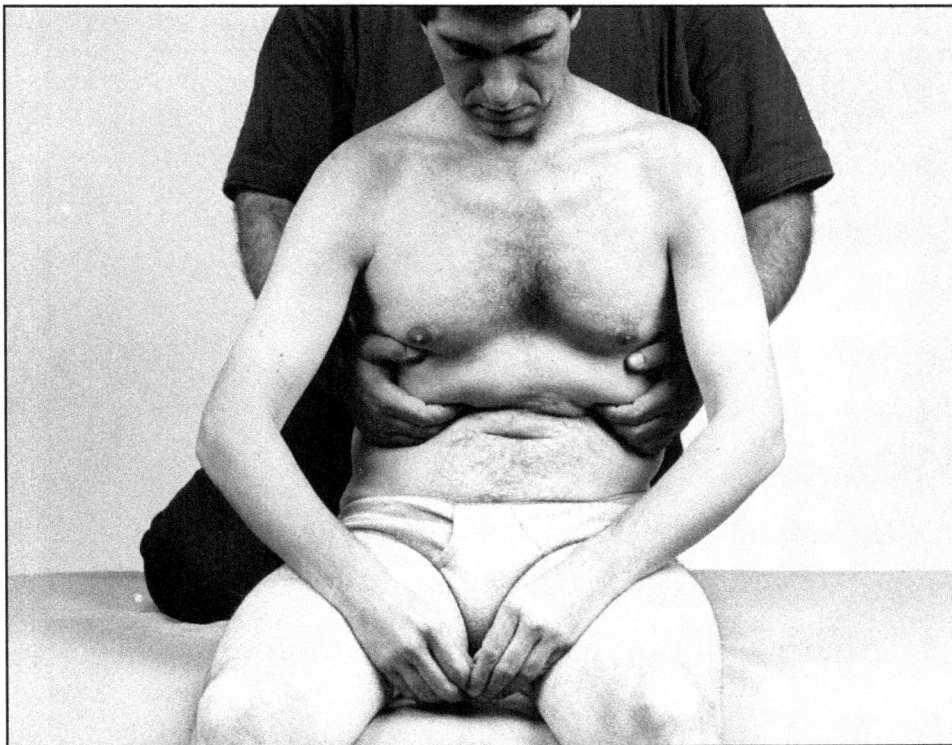

Seated Lower Costal Cage Treatment

4. **Upper Thoracic Treatment, Patient Supine Using an Indirect Technique**

Operator sits at the side of the patient with one hand underneath and one hand above, contacting the upper thoracic cage. **Assessment** should be made of the relative compliance to compression and the general feeling of tension of the thoracic wall.

Treatment should be applied by introducing directions of ease between the two palpating hands (lateral translation, superior/inferior translation, rotation, side-bending, inhalation/exhalation, and compression). Only relatively small amounts of these movements need to be introduced in order to begin the unwinding process of this technique. Hand contact should be light, and when the unwinding is completed, the tissue should be reassessed.

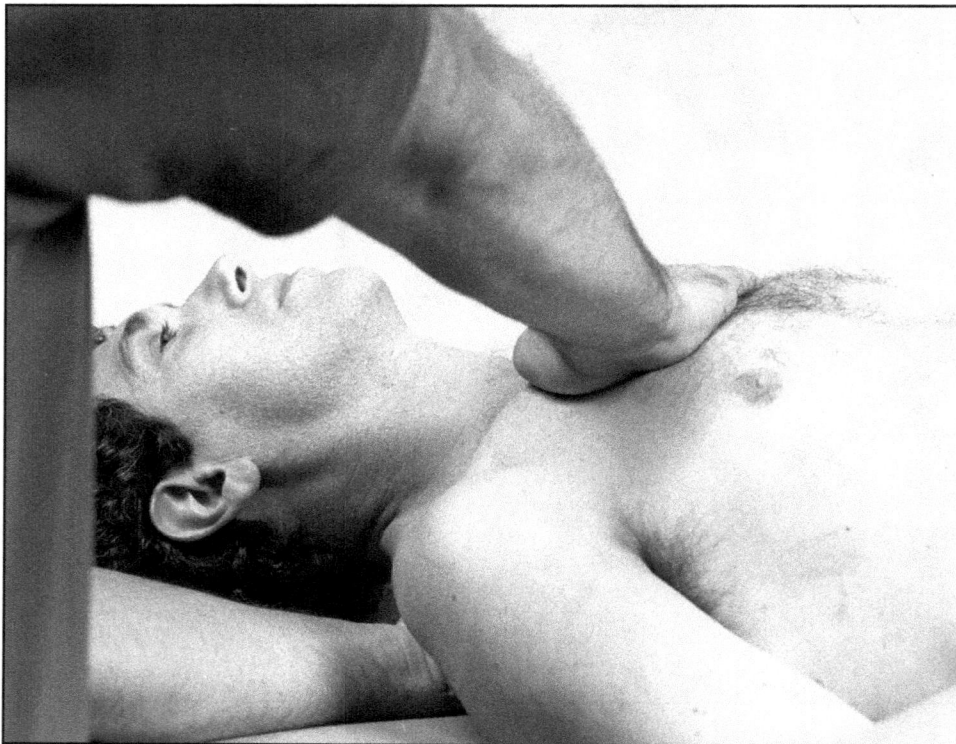

Supine Upper Thoracic Cage Treatment
Horizontal Approach

14

5. **Upper Thoracic Release, Patient Supine Using a Direct Technique**

For **assessment**, the operator stands at the head of the table and places either hand into the region of the patient's sternum and applies a compressive force posteriorly and inferiorly to test the complicance of the sternal region.

For **treatment**, pressure is maintained and inhalation resisted until the next exhalation allows for further compressive force to follow into the tissues under the treating hand. This compressive force should be maintained until there is a sense of melting away of the myofascial restriction or there is a sense of an unwinding which may occur briefly in a curvilinear path. This treatmernt can be perfomed with one or two hands. The two-handed technique would contact the costal cage just lateral to the sternum on either side. Reassess after treatment.

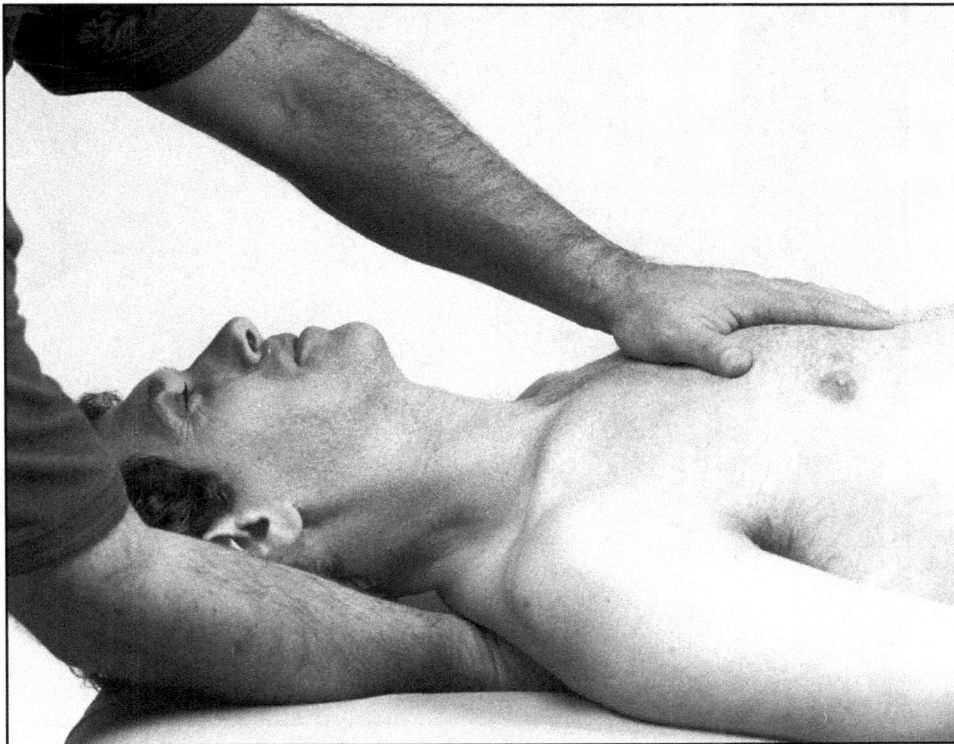

Supine Upper Thoracic Cage Treatment
Vertical Approach

15

6. Upper Thoracic Release, Patient Supine Using a Direct Stretch Technique

Operator sits at the head of the table and places both hands posteriorly underneath the patient's thorax approximately midway down the thoracic spine, extending the fingers all the way to the thoracolumbar junction if necessary. Relative tension is **assessed** in these paraspinal areas, extending into the three-dimensional structures of the entire thoracic cage.

For **treatment**, an area of maximal restriction is determined and used as a point of entry. Direct stretch is applied in a cephalad and lateral direction, applying some anterior translation as well. This stretch is held until there is a sense of loosening of the tissues underneath the hands and tissue returns to a point of balance, after which it is reassessed.

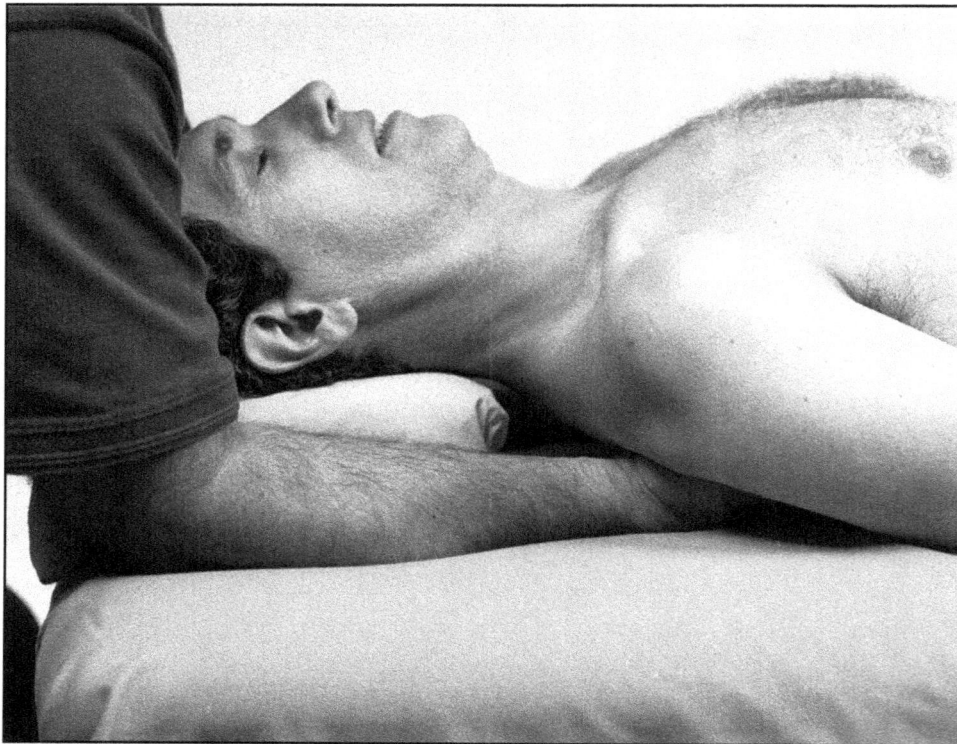

Supine Thoracic Spine Treatment

7. Scapulothoracic Release, Patient Side-Lying Using an Indirect Technique

The operator stands on the side of the table, facing the patient at a point about equal with his shoulder. Patient is side-lying perpendicular to the table at the edge closest to the operator. The operator's caudad arm is brought underneath the patient's arm and finds the medial and lateral border of the scapula under which the fingers and thumb rests. The opposite hand comes around from the top and finds the medial border, and both hands have contact simultaneosuly. **Assessment** is made of the relative gliding restriction of the scapula in superior/inferior, lateral translation left/right, and rotation clockwise/counterclockwise movements to determine the directions of greatest ease. The scapula is positioned in these three directions of ease, while at the same time the operator pins the patient's shoulder between his palpating hands and his chest.

For **treatment**, these positions of ease are held until there is a release that occurs and is followed until the tissues come to a new point of balance and rest. A second phase of this treatment requires that the operator's caudad hand is repositioned underneath the inferior tip of the patient's scapula. The movement of the scapula is similarly reassessed and an indirect technique again applied and the release followed. At the end of these two releases, the overall motion should be reassessed and an improvement in balance determined.

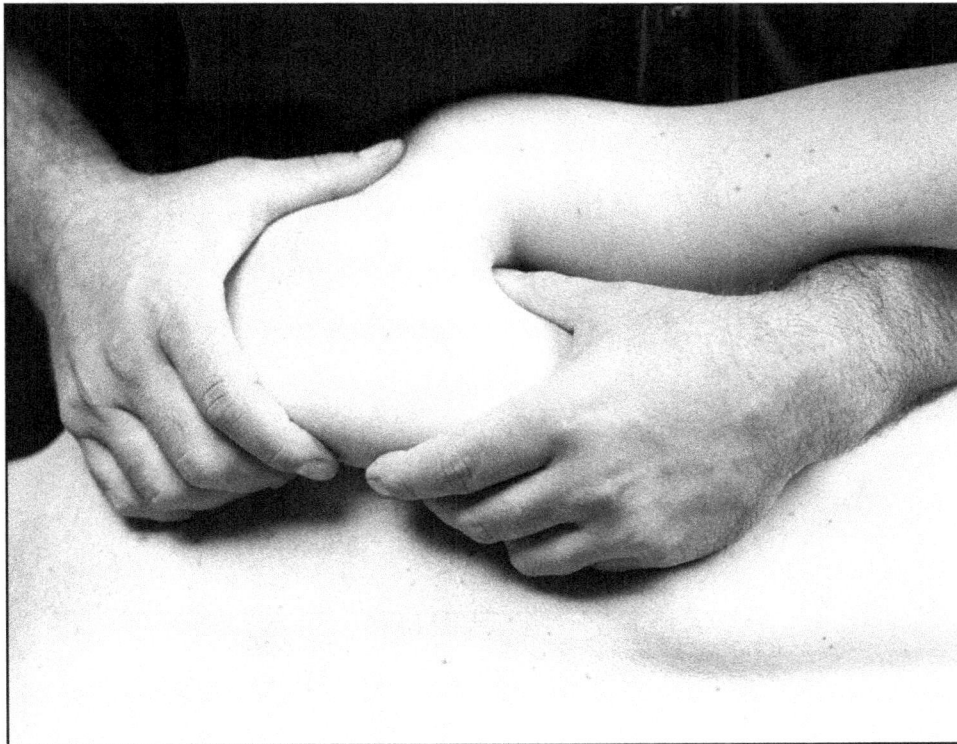

Sidelying Scapulothoracic Treatment
Arm Adducted

8. Scapulothoracic Release, Patient Side-Lying Using a Direct Unwinding Technique

The operator stands as before. For **assessment**, he brings the patient's arm into flexion, the operator's cephalward arm underneath the patient's arm and around the back of the scapula, contacting the medial border. The operator's other hand contacts the medial border of the scapula from below.

For **treatment**, directions of ease and resistance are tested similarly as in the previous exercise and the scapulothoracic unit is held in the direction of resistance into the barrier until an unwinding occurs. The unwinding is followed until it comes to rest, at which time motions are reassessed for greater symmetry.

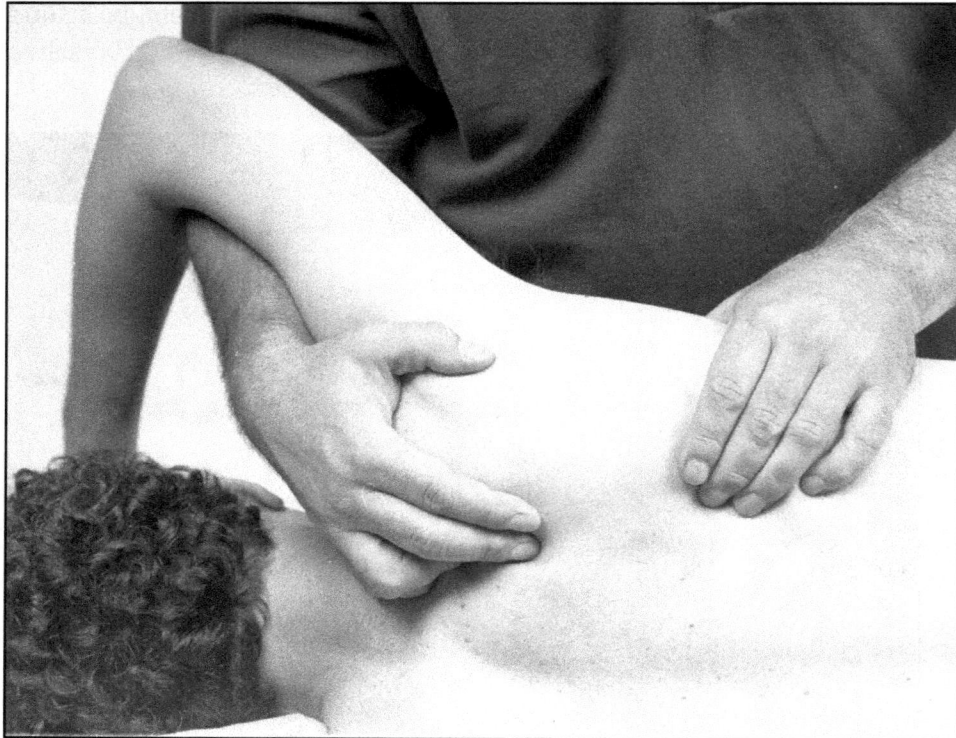

Sidelying Scapulothoracic Treatment
Arm Abducted

9. Upper Anterior Costal Cage Release, Patient Supine Using a Direct Pumping Technique

Operator stands at the patient's side, facing the patient with both hands over the upper anterior costal cage at about the level of the 2nd and 3rd ribs. **Assessment** is made of the relative compliance of the left versus the right costal cage component, and a direct pumping technique is used by compressing the side that is relatively loose and by gently, rhythmically pumping the side that is tight in a posterior direction, i.e. into the table.

Treatment is continued with a slow pumping rhythm until there is a sense of softening of the myofascial tensions in the entire thoracic outlet region. A feeling of increased force transference between the hands will occur from the pumping motion induced. This increase in force transference relflects a release of the myofascial tensions. Reassessment after treatment is mandatory.

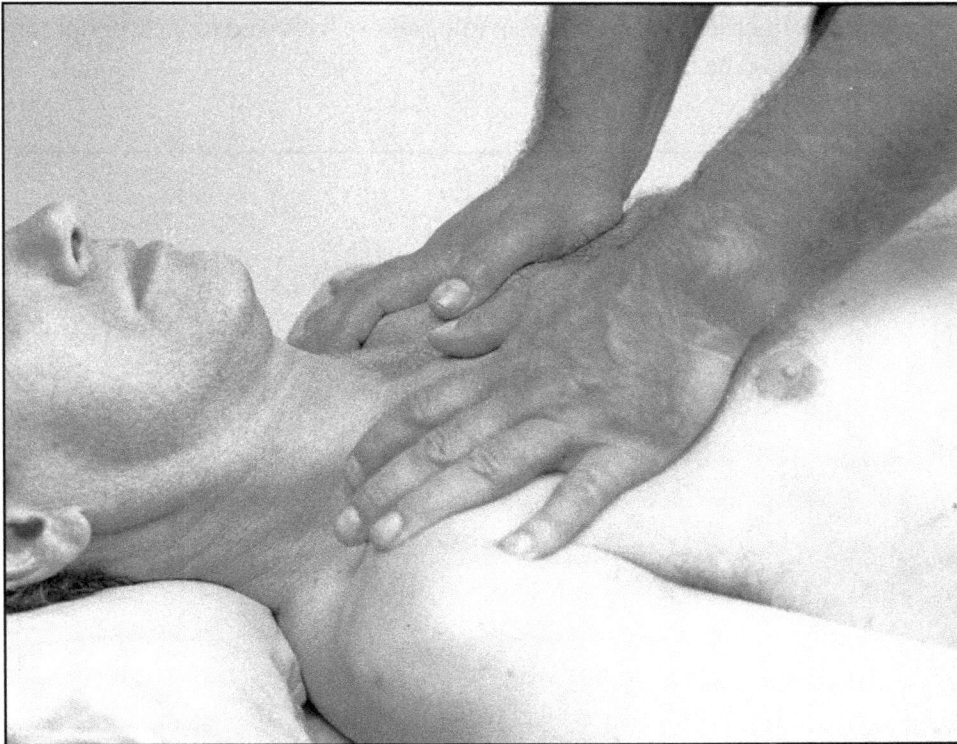

Supine Upper Costal Cage Treatment

10. Cervicothoracic Junction Release, Patient Supine Using a Direct Unwinding Technique

Operator sits at the patient's head with each hand over the superior aspect of the coastal cage atop the 1st rib. The heels of the hands should be contacting just over the trapezius border, and the fingers contacting the lateral aspects of the scalene muscles and rest slightly anterior and inferior to the clavicle. The thumbs should come posteriorly around the transverse processes to the vertebral body of T2. From this position, the operator should **assess** the relative compliance of the tissues in response to an inferior force applied alternately by each hand into the thoracic cage, left then right. Relative compliance and restriction of each side should be determined, and a positioning of the thoracic cage into the barrier should ensue.

To initiate **treatment**, additional positions of restriction should be added, testing anterior/posterior compliance (i.e. rotation) of left to right costal cage components, lateral and AP translation of the entire thoracic cage, as well as changes in the patient's head position to increase positioning into the restrictive barrier (e.g. head rotation left). Positions of resistance should be added together to give a cumulative "necklace" effect, while any inherent releases are followed to their endpoint. Reassess tissue compliance following the treatment.

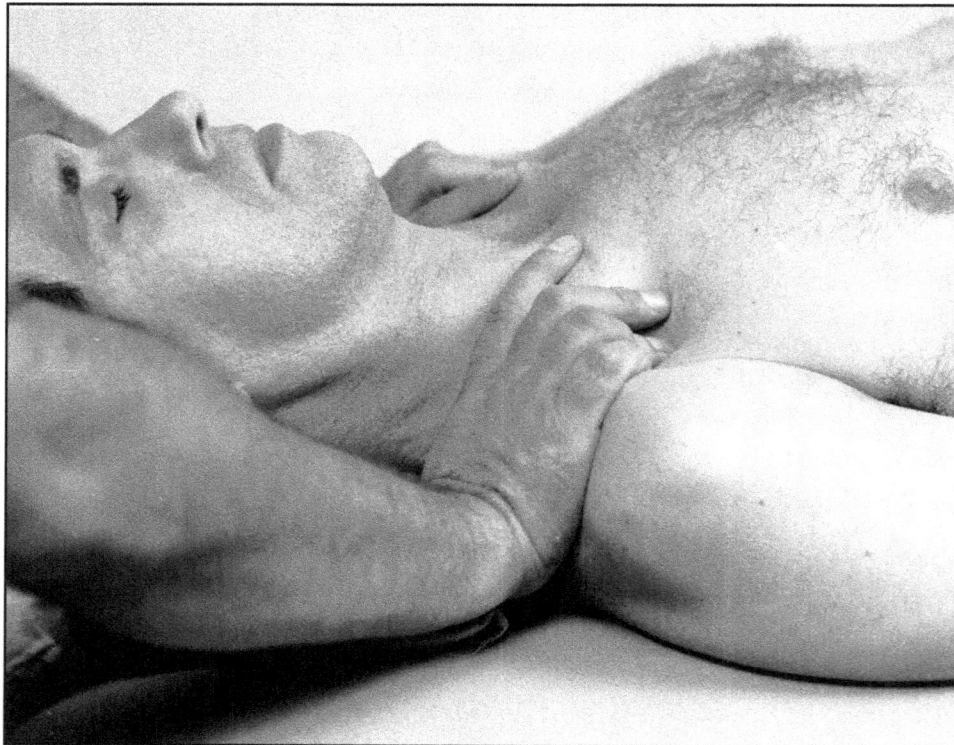

Supine Cervicothoracic Treatment
Clavicular Contact

MYOFASCIAL TREATMENT
OF THE LOWER EXTREMITY

1. Ankle Treatment, Patient Supine Using an Indirect Technique

Assessment is made by gently inverting and everting the talus joint of the ankle. Relative compliance and restriction should be assessed and the ankle positioned slightly in the direction of ease or greater compliance to initiate **treatment**. Additional movements in the ankle should be tested for directions of compliance which should be added to the first one already applied (e.g. dorsiflexion/plantarflexion, anterior/posterior glide, forefoot pronation/supination). All these directions should be applied simultaneously and the unwinding of the tissues sensed and followed within moments after indirect positioning is attained. This unwinding should be followed through its release in the ankle and palpated all the way to the knee, hip, and pelvis as well. Reassessment of eversion and inversion should be made at the end of the treatment.

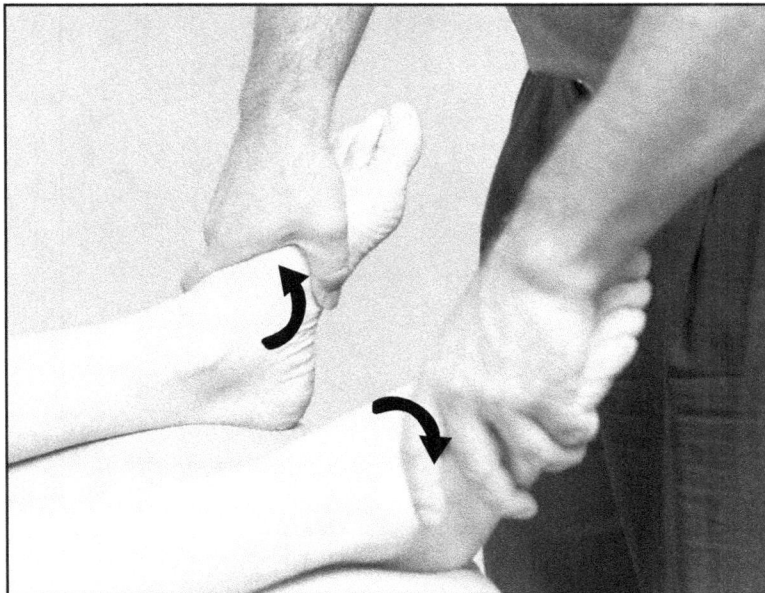

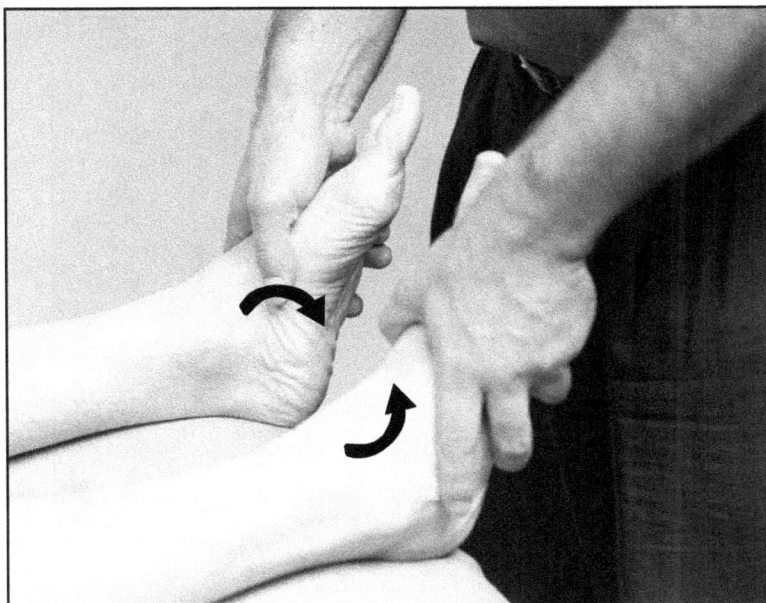

Ankle Assessment: Eversion and Inversion

2. Knee Treatment Supine Using a Direct Stretch Technique

The knee is **assessed** while extended flat on the table, and the tibial tuberosity is located and compared with the patella to see that it lies somewhere in the midline of the patella. If the tibial tuberosity lies medial or lateral to this imagined midline, then this knee should be treated with the following technique.

The knee is **treated** flexed with the foot flat on the table and the knee is gently translated medially with one hand, while the other hand stabilizes the foot on the table by holding the ankle. The slack is taken out of the mechanism in a medial direction until a sense of the barrier is achieved. At this point, the barrier should be held, and as the barrier eases, the knee should be moved further in the medial direction until a sense of melting of the barrier occurs. Reassessment after treatment should follow to see if the tibial tuberosity has been shifted.

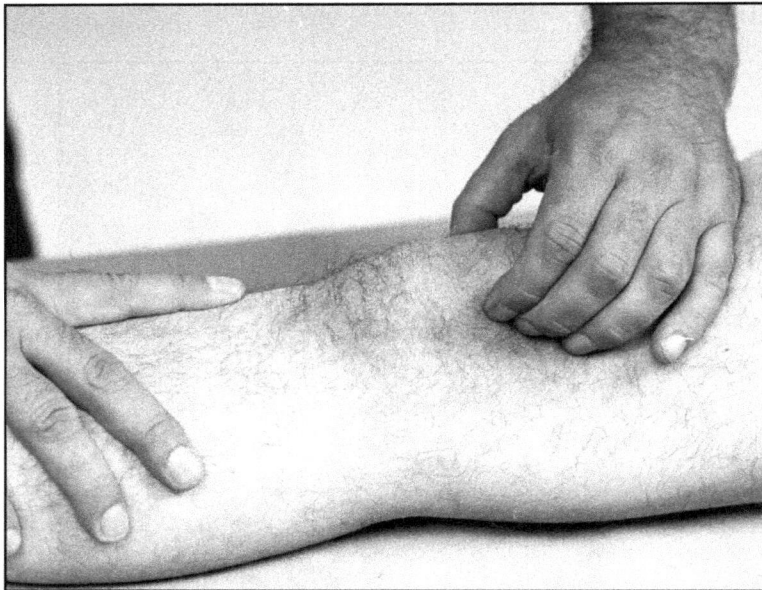

Tibial Assessment

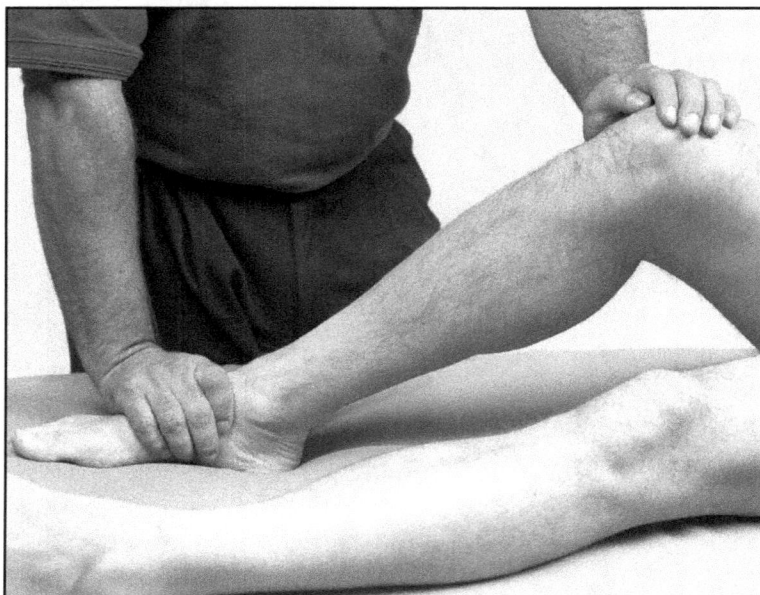

Knee Treatment

22

3. Single Lower Extremity Release, Patient Supine Using a Direct Unwinding Technique

The lower extremity should be contacted for **assessment** by placing one hand underneath the Achilles tendon and the other hand over the dorsal aspect of the forefoot. Traction should be applied into the entire lower extremity by fully dorsiflexing and everting the foot while gently leaning backwards. In this position, tension in the total cylindrical mechanism of the lower extremity and pelvis should be assessed. Likewise, the same procedure should be applied to the opposite leg and the leg of greatest restriction or tension should be chosen to treat. Bilateral assessment can also be carried out as shown.

Treatment involves resuming the same position of assessment while fine tuning with engagement of the barrier in hip flexion/extension, abduction/adduction, and internal/external rotation. Hold this position until the tissues in the entire lower extremity cylinder begin to unwind. The sense of unwinding may project all the way into the hip, sacroiliac and even lumbosacral spine, and this release may cause various movement at all the joints in between. These movements should be slowly followed by the operator through their arcing curvilinear releases (e.g. knee flexion, hip abduction and flexion moving into hip adduction and extension, with knee extension). This release may take several arcing cycles before coming to a point of balance, at which time the cylindrical mechanism of the lower extremities should be reassessed for a change in tension.

If the unwinding is not felt, the operator may gently lead by introducing directions of ease, then following the patient's response. Alternating the leading and following will be like a dance, eventually blurring the distinction as it all happens at once.

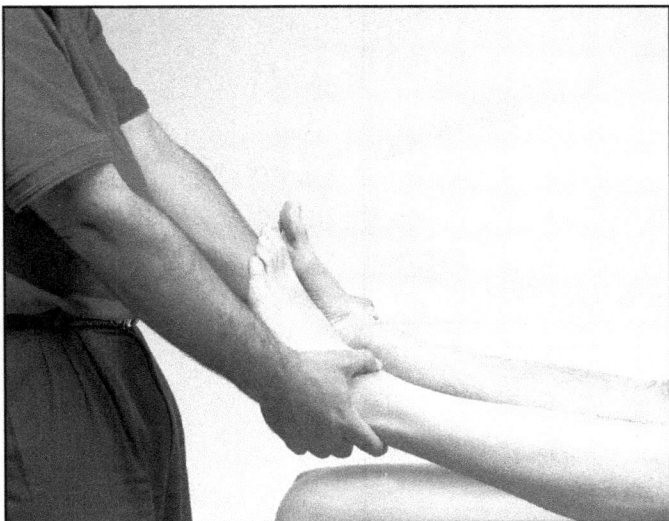

Bilateral Lower Extremity
Traction Assessment

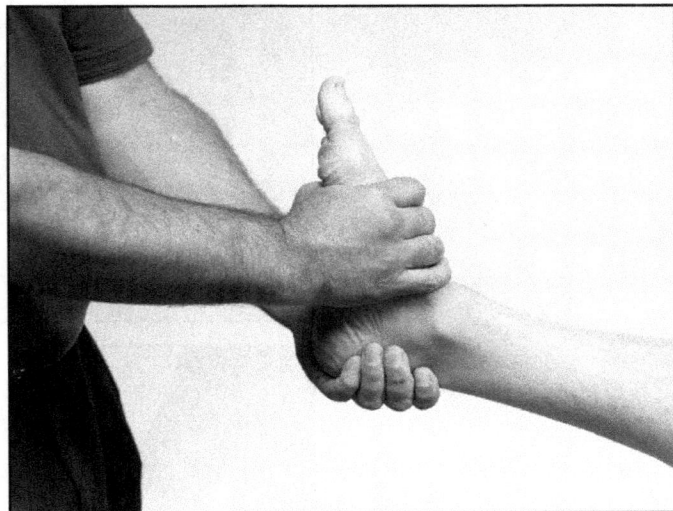

Unilateral Lower Extremity
Traction Assessment

(Continued ...)

3. Single Lower Extremity Release, Patient Supine Using a Direct Unwinding Technique (Continued)

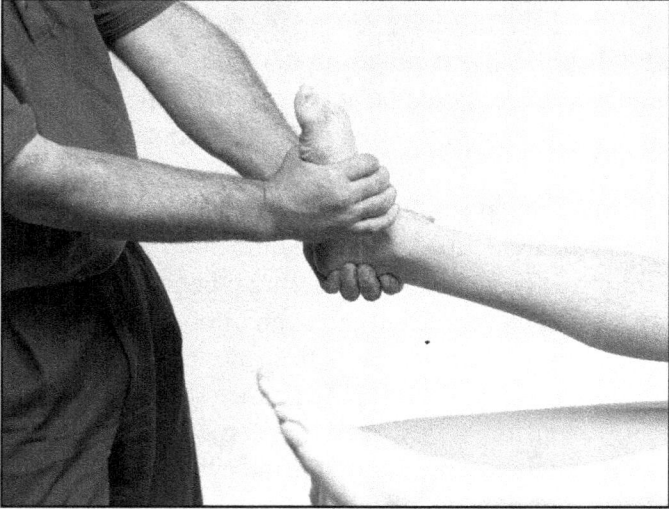

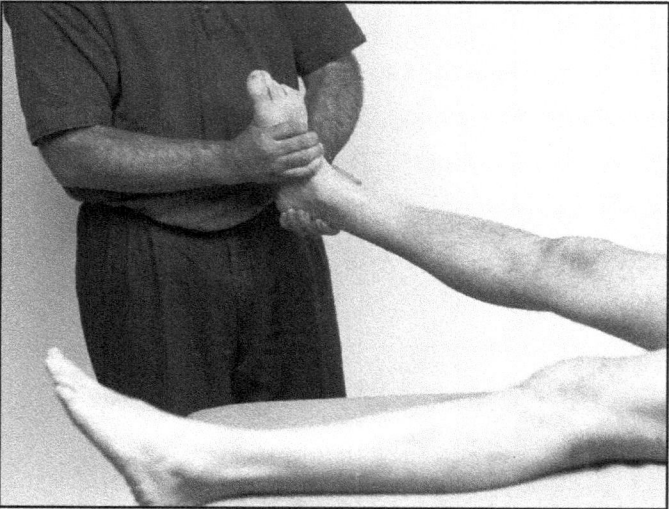

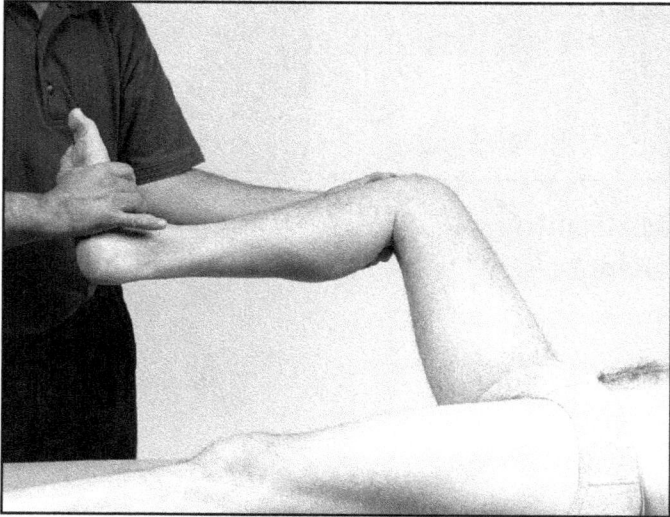

3. Single Lower Extremity Release, Patient Supine Using a Direct Unwinding Technique (Continued)

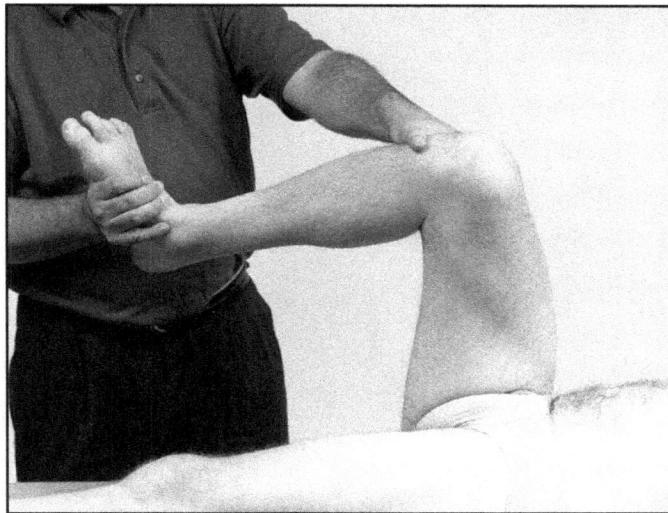

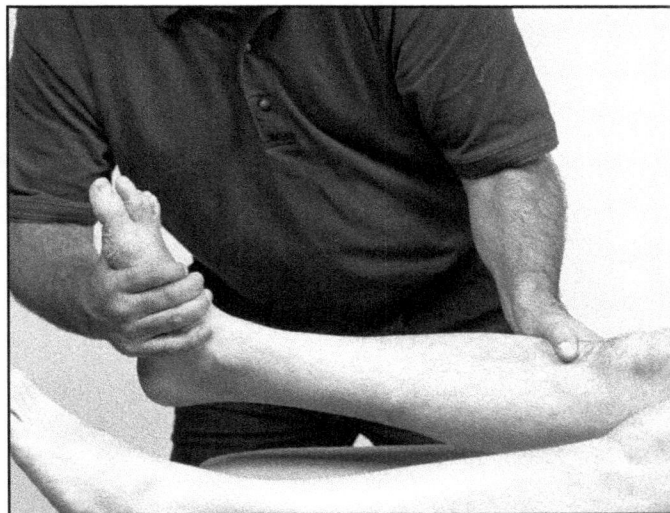

Notes

MYOFASCIAL TREATMENT
OF THE UPPER EXTREMITY

1. Treatment of the Finger by Using an Indirect Technique

An area of pain or dysfunction of the finger and any of its joints can be **assessed** as follows. The soft tissues around the joint focus are held proximally with one hand, while the other hands holds the distal portion of the digit. Motion testing is carried out in all possible directions, lateral translation, superior/inferior translation, rotation, side-bending, and flexion/extension. Compression and distraction are also tested.

After these are assessed, they are then **treated** by combining them all in their direction of ease and waiting for a release to occur of the myofascial and even articular tissues involved. The unwinding is followed until it comes to a stop. Sometimes the release will extend from the finger into the wrist, elbow, and shoulder areas. These releases require more focus on effects further away from the point of treatment; however, with practice they can become routine. After treatment, motion testing is carried out to reassess.

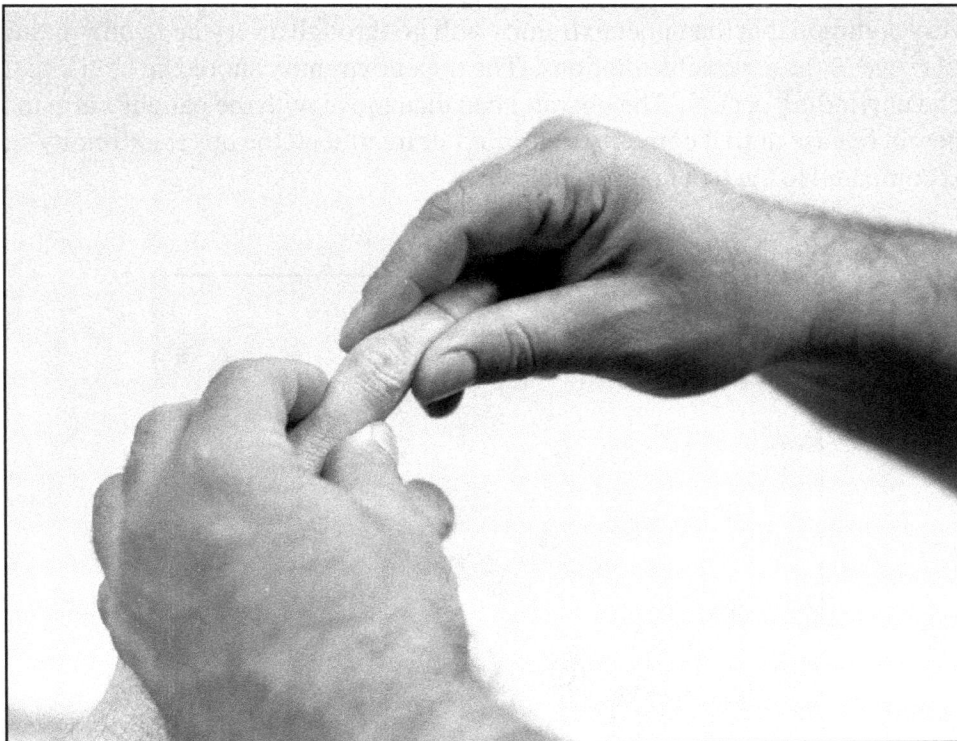

Finger Treatment

2. Single and Double Upper Extremity Treatment, Patient Supine Using a Direct Unwinding Technique

The operator stands to the side of the patient, contacting both of the patient's forearms as they are oriented to the patient's side. The side of the restricted upper extremity is **assessed** by use of either a gentle traction test into the shoulders alternately or by means of visual observation or any other means that is acceptable to the operator. If a traction test is used through the forearms, usually the side of restriction will recruit movement at the neck and head before the other side. This is due to the increased myofascial tension in the cylindrical mechanism. Treatment can be performed with the one extremity alone or with both extremities simultaneously.

Single extremity treatment involves one of the operator's hands holding onto the patient's elbow, palm facing upwards underneath the elbow. The operator's thumb should rest approximately on the proximal radial head, with a slight twist directed in a pronating fashion. The other hand contacts the patient's wrist and furthers the pronation twist to the endpoint, applying gentle tension into the tissue with traction between the two hands. The position or point of greatest restriction should be determined by taking the arm and slightly adjusting the angle in forward flexion/extension, abduction/adduction to determine the point at which to begin treatment. The position of the operator can be shifted slightly to enhance this focus on the point of entry. The operator can stand on the opposite side from the patient's extremity or can stand at the head and bring the shoulder into extreme flexion. In treating the upper extremity in this manner, it is very common that the upper extremity will go through a very large unwinding, which will include the full range of these possible motions. The upper extremity should be held into these direct barriers until the unwinding occurs. The operator can then move with the patient's arm to follow closely behind the inherent release until it comes to a stop. After treatment, the upper extremity should be reassessed and compared to the other one, as before.

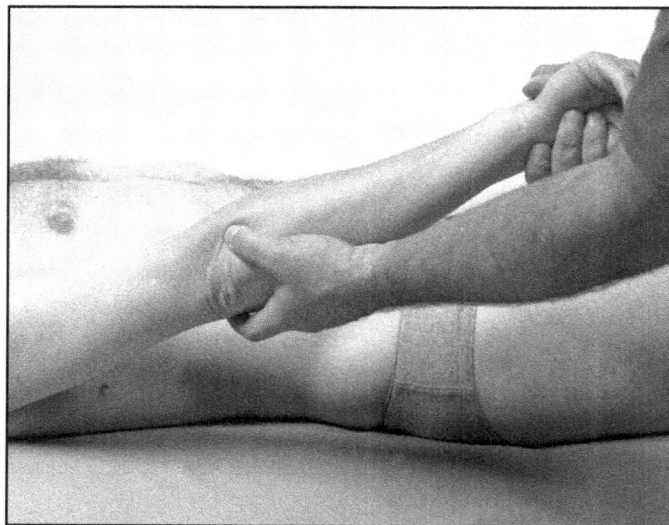

Single Upper Extremity Treatment

2. Double Upper Extremity Treatment, Patient Supine Using a Direct Unwinding Technique

Double upper extremity treatment involves treatment of both upper extremities together, positioning each upper extremity in a position of relative restriction (relative due to the limitation of having to contact both upper extremities at once without letting go). This technique is often used with the operator standing at the patient's head with both arms in full flexion overhead. The operator shifts from side to side to determine the myofascial restriction of the upper extremity through its attachment into the upper thoracic spine and rib cage. Treatment with the double extremity contact often involves a direct stretch, with only minimal unwinding occuring. Significant unwinding can occur, however, and the operator should be prepared to follow a large unwinding with a double extremity technique. (Contact of both extremities is through the forearms or wrists. Care must be taken not to cause the patient discomfort with this handhold.)

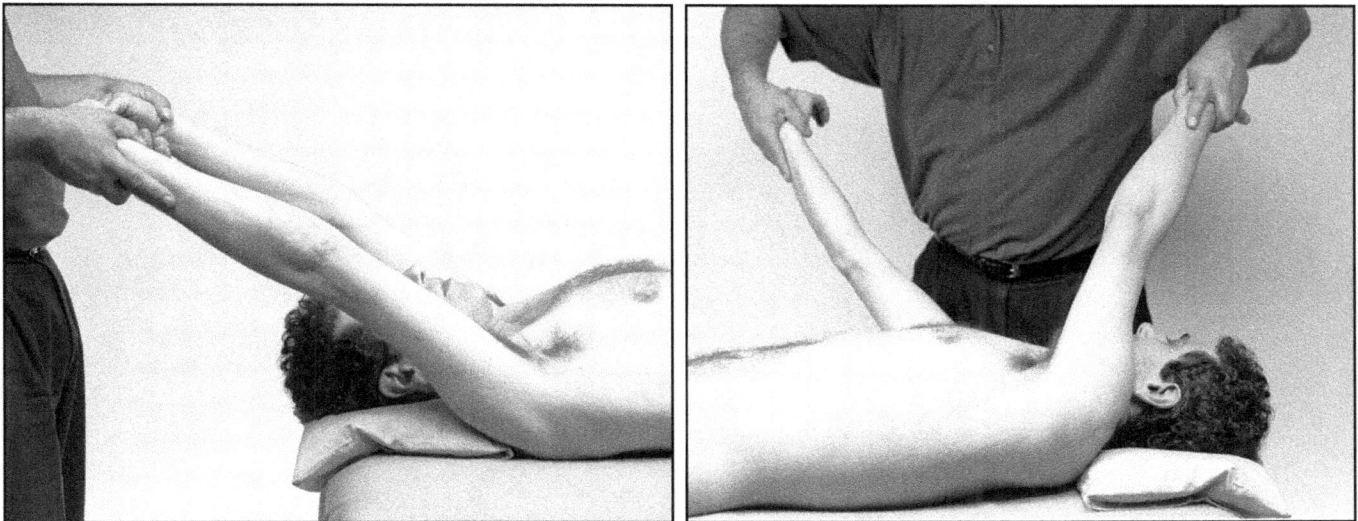

Double Upper Extremity Treatment

Notes

TREATMENT OF THE CERVICAL SPINE

1. Cervicothoracic Twist, Patient Supine Using a Direct Stretching Technique

The operator stands at the head of the table with hands contacting the patient's neck. **Assess** the tension of the tissues in the cervicothoracic and cervical area posteriorly, laterally, and anteriorly to test their relative myofascial tensions.

Assessment is followed by **treatment**, where the operator places his knee behind the neck of the patient while lifting the patient's head with a posterior hold around the patient's mid-upper cervical region. Either hand can be used. This upper contact point maintains a moderate flexing traction, while the other hand contacts the upper thoracic spine to take the traction in the opposite direction. Twist is then introduced between the two hands, rotating the head either left or right in the direction of the barrier. The barrier is engaged and held, with moderate-to-extreme traction force awaiting the melting away and myofascial release that occurs between the two hands. This treatment involves mostly a viscoelastic stretch release, and unwinding is minimal, due to the hand positioning. After the treatment, the tissue should be reassessed as described.

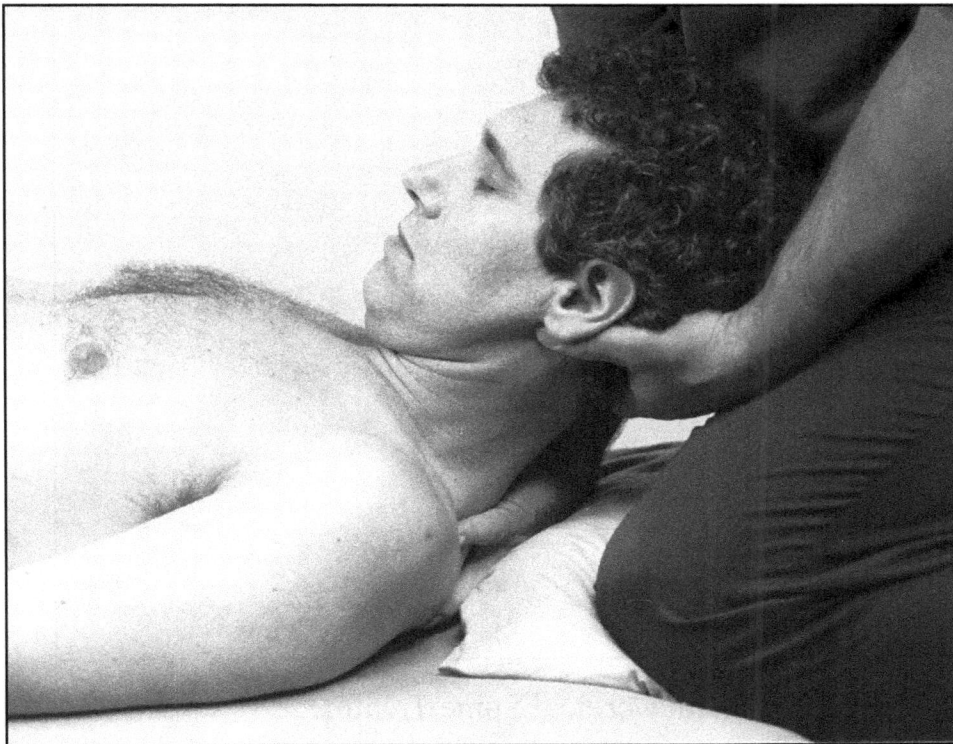

Supine Cervicothoracic Treatment
Head Contact

2. <u>Lateral Cervical Spine Treatment,</u>
<u>Patient Supine Using an Indirect Unwinding Technique</u>

The operator sits at the head of the patient with hands on either side of the cervical spine overlying the sternomastoid and scalene muscle bellies, tension is **assessed** with light compression and initial motion introduced, including flexion, extension, rotation, side-bending, compression, distraction, and lateral and AP translation as well. These forces are introduced only through the soft tissue complex, with only slight initiation of facet motion.

For **treatment**, The summation of all of these directions of ease is combined and the indirect unwinding follows until there is a melting away of myofascial tension and the release comes to a stop. After treatment is completed, the tissue should be reassessed and motion tested to assure greater balance.

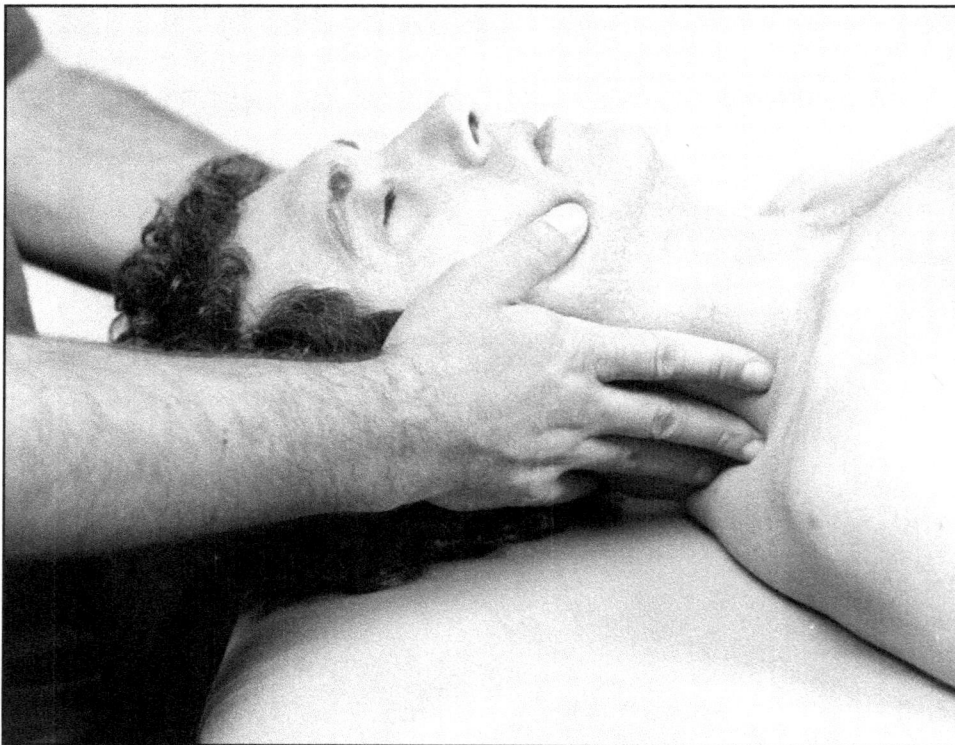

Lateral Cervical Spine Treatment

3. Cervicothoracic Junction, Patient Seated Using an Indirect Technique

This technique is similar to the upper costal cage technique with the patient supine, where we did a direct unwinding technique. There is similar hand contact over the apex of the costal cage, fingers forward over the clavicle, thumb in back behind the transverse process of T2. Tensions are **assessed** through motion testing of side-bending, rotation, flexion and extension. Additional levers may be used by positioning the patient's head forward or backward, the arms up or down, depending on which brings more ease into the tissues. (Frequently, with car accidents, it is a good technique to ask the patient to assume the driving position with hands on an imaginary steering wheel, allowing his body to move in ways which may reproduce the moment of injury.)

Treatment reproduction of this moment of trauma stimulates an inherent myofascial release which should be followed and may go through a large range of motion in an arcing curvilinear release. At the completion of the unwinding, the patient should be reassessed to see if thoracic outlet motion testing has improved.

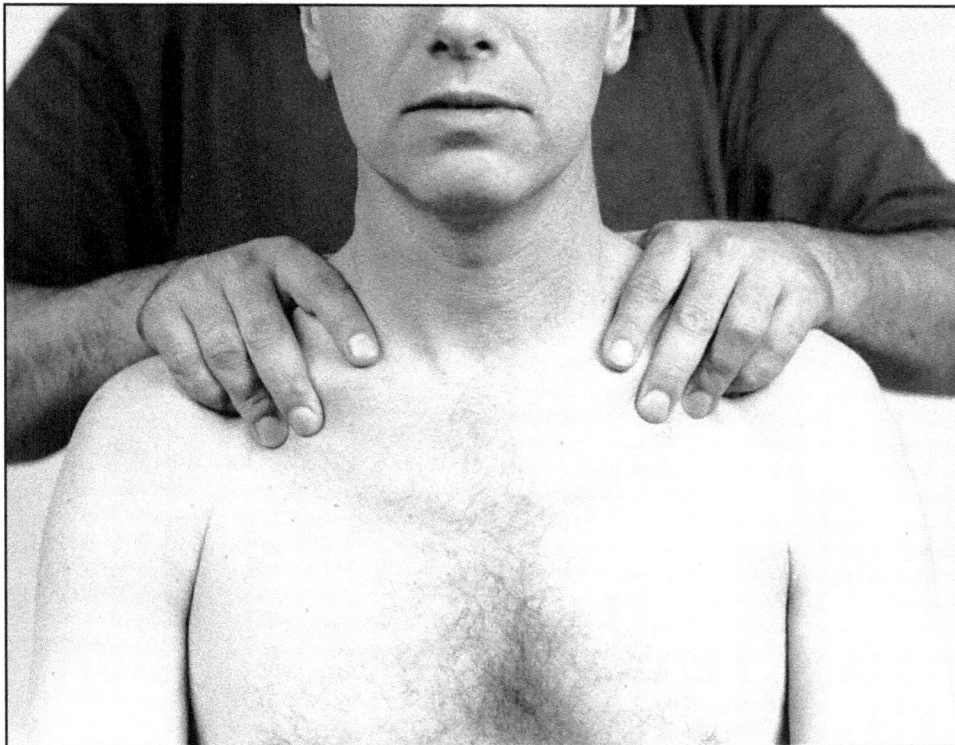

Seated Cervicothoracic Treatment

Notes

LUMBOSACRAL SPINE AND PELVIS

1. Lumbosacral Spine, Patient Prone Using a Direct Unwinding Technique, Direct Pumping Technique, and Direct Stretching Technique

Assessment. The patient is prone. The operator stands at the patient's side facing towards the feet. The operators cephalad hand contacts the patient's mid lumbar spine, the other hand contacting the sacrum, with the heel of the hand on the sacral base and the fingers falling inferiorly over the sacral apex. The other hand should be oriented similarly and traction created between the two hands to assess lumbosacral mobility. Sacral compression should also be carried out with both hands over the sacrum, one on top of the other, assessing anterior compliance.

Treatment is an extension of assessment wherein the traction is maintained in an arcing manner, with the sacral contact likened to contact on a sphere where the force is up and over the edge of the sphere represented by the sacral curve. This traction should be held, an unwinding will occur, and the lumbosacral components may rotate in opposite directions, with side-bending coupled as well. Follow the release until it comes to a still point, at which time the lumbosacral mobility should be reassessed.

A **direct pumping technique** may be used, wherein the hand position on the sacrum is the same but the other hand comes and rests on top of the sacral hand in a perpendicular manner, the two hands forming a cross. Direct pumping through the sacral apex causing the sacral base to come posteriorly should be performed in a slow and rhythmic fashion. The barrier should be engaged with each pump and then gently released and contacted again repeatedly until there is a melting away of myofascial tension on the lumbosacral area.

Using the same handhold, a **direct stretch** may be accomplished by slightly shifting the focus into the heel of the hand, pushing the sacral base anteriorly and inferiorly and holding for a direct myofascial release.

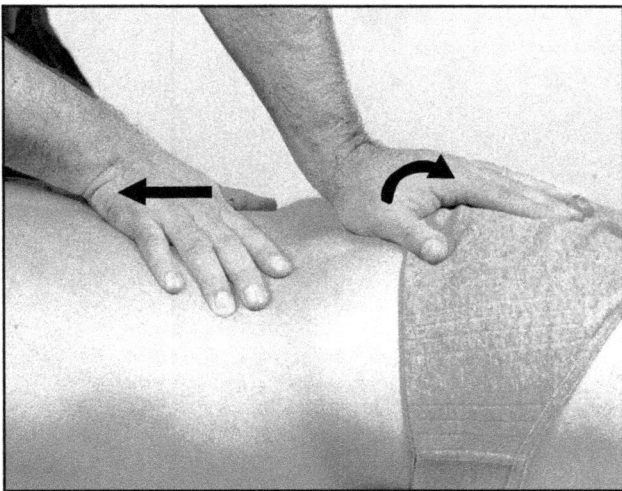

Prone Lumbosacral Spine
Assessment and Treatment

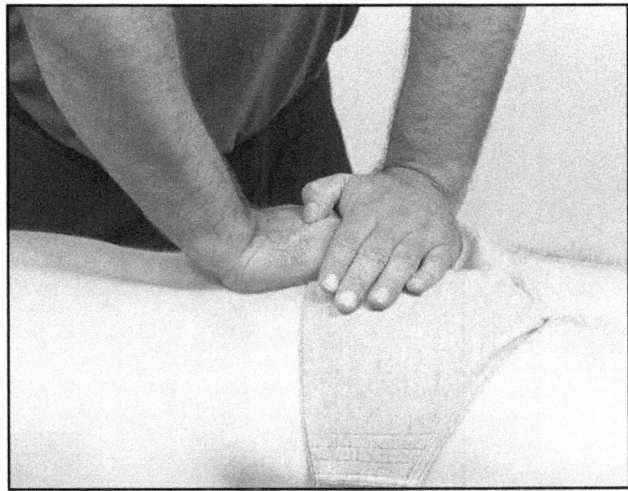

Prone Sacral Assessment
and Treatment

2. Treatment of the Pelvis, Patient Prone Using a Direct Stretching, Direct Pumping, and Indirect Unwinding Technique

The operator stands to the side of the patient, facing his upper back and head. Contact is made bilaterally over the pelvis by placing the thumbs just medial to the PSIS, with the thenar eminences falling lateral to the lateral angles of the sacrum, the majority of the hand falling into the lateral gluteal and piriformis region, and the fingers falling laterally towards the hip and iliac crest. From this position, pelvic musculature and ligaments can be **assessed** with alternating compression into the table, left to right, side-bending, and lateral translation to determine the directions of restriction.

Treatment can be performed by engaging the barriers and holding the entire pelvic mechanism into its three-dimensional barrier and held there until a sense of unwinding occurs, at which point the tissues should be followed until they come to a rest. Some lateral tracton can be applied to further stimulate this release similar to the technique performed at the thoracolumbar junction with the patient prone. Tissue should be reassessed after treatment.

The same technique can be applied using a **pumping technique**, with the loose side being held compressed into the table and the tight side pumped with a gentle rhythmic anterior compression. Some superior or inferior vector can be added, whichever is the direction of restriction. Gentle pumping should be carried out until a sense of loosening of the myofascial mechanism is palpated. Retesting after treatment is suggested.

An alternate **indirect unwinding technique** can be performed by the three-point contact technique. The focus of this technique is in the placement of the thumbs on the sacrotuberous ligaments bilaterally, The index fingers then fall into the sacral sulcus, and the middle finger falls into the gluteal tissue laterally. Motion between the sides of the pelvis can be assessed by introducing caudal/cephalad shearing and anterior-posterior rotation. Treatment is then begun by positioning in the direction of ease and allowing the tissue to unwind. Reassessment afterwards is essential.

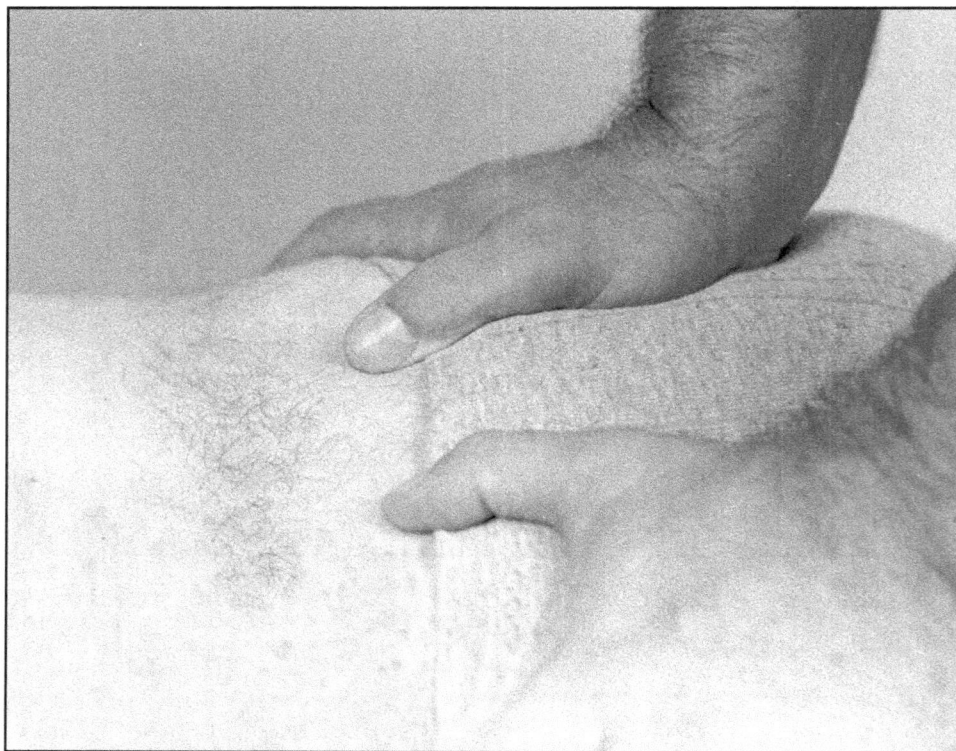

Prone Pelvis Assessment

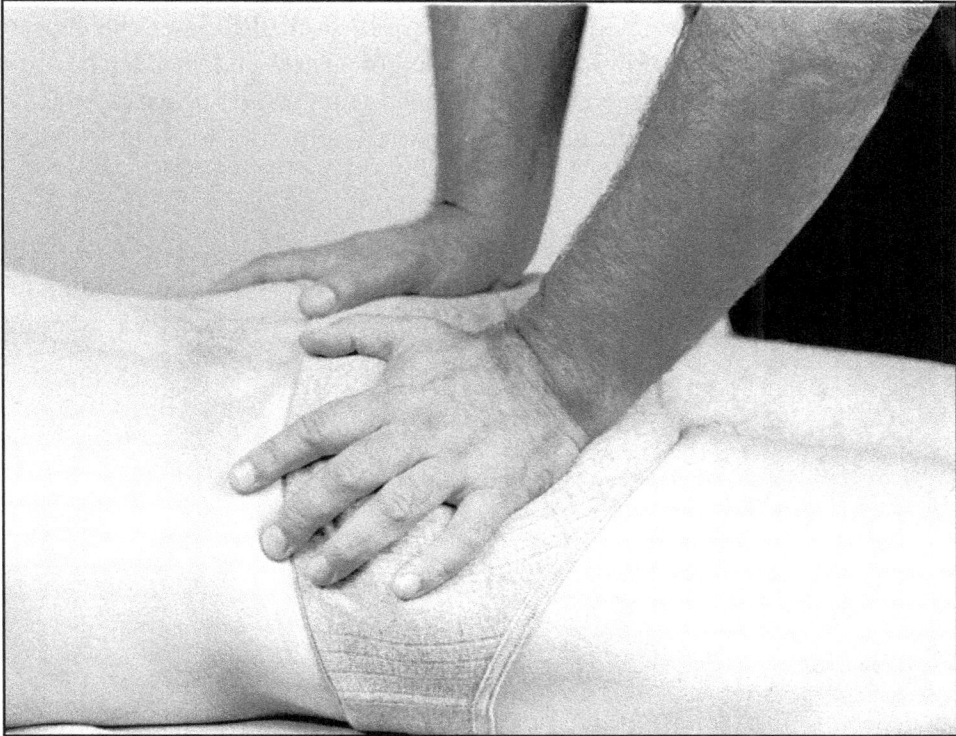
Prone Pelvis Treatment

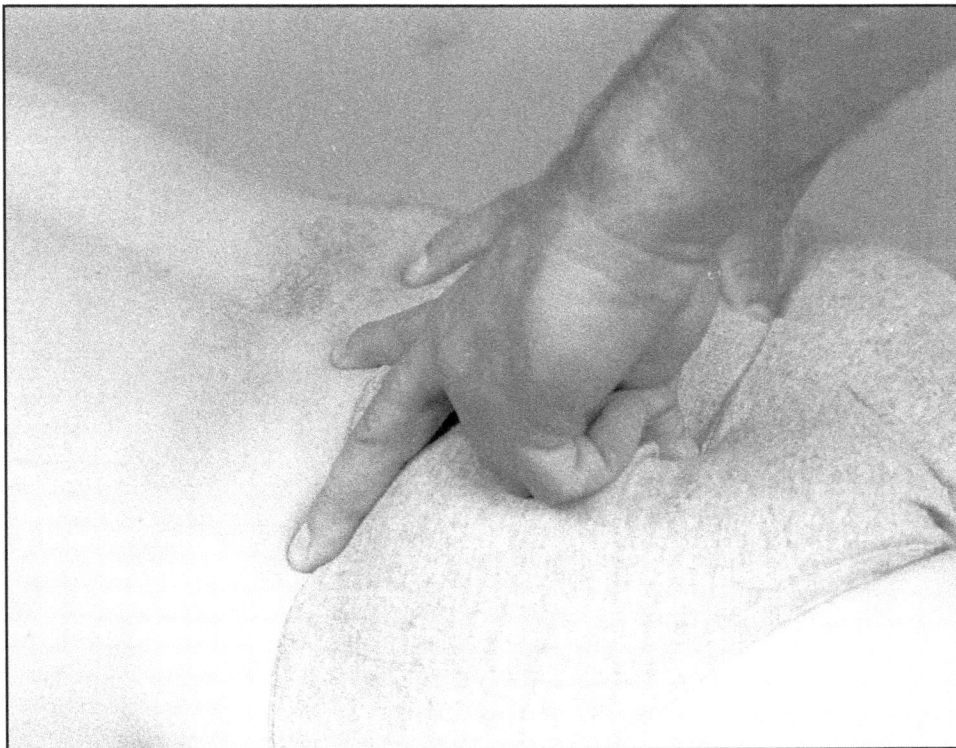
Prone Pelvis Treatment
Three Point Contact

3. Pelvic Treatment, Patient Supine Using Direct Stretching Technique and a Direct Pumping Technique

The patient's bilateral ASIS are contacted in a similar fashion as the PSIS with the thumbs medial to the bone and the rest of the hand falling inferiorly over the inguinal area and the deep pelvic musculature including the psoas muscle. Again, three-dimensional symmetry should be **assessed** using rotation, side-bending, translation and carrying the hemipelvis towards anterior and posterior rotation into their respective barriers.

For **treatment**, the barriers should be held and a slight lateral traction added to stimulate myofascial release. Alternately, the same technique with a **pumping** action may be used, holding the tissues on the loose side and pumping the tissues on the tight side into the barriers, as previously described. After treatment, tissues should be reassessed for greater symmetry.

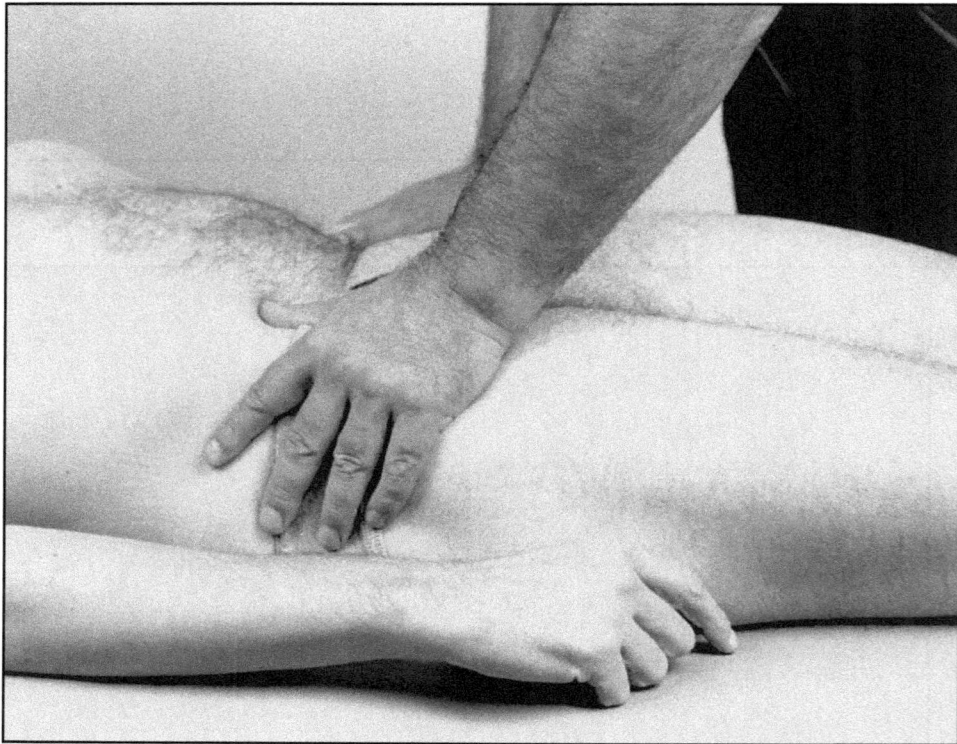

Supine Pelvis Treatment

4. Pubic Fascial Release, Patient Supine Using a Direct Stretching Technique

The operator stands to the side of the patient facing his head, with his hands contacting the pubic symphysis. Behind the pubic symphysis there are ligamentous and tendonous attachments originating from the inguinal and abdominal components. The tension is **assessed** just posterior to the pubic symphisis in an inferior direction.

Treatment is carried out by just increasing the stretch slowly, asking the patient to breathe deeply, and with each exhalation the tension is increased until a sensation of melting away of this fascial restriction is appreciated. Reassessment after treatment is suggested.

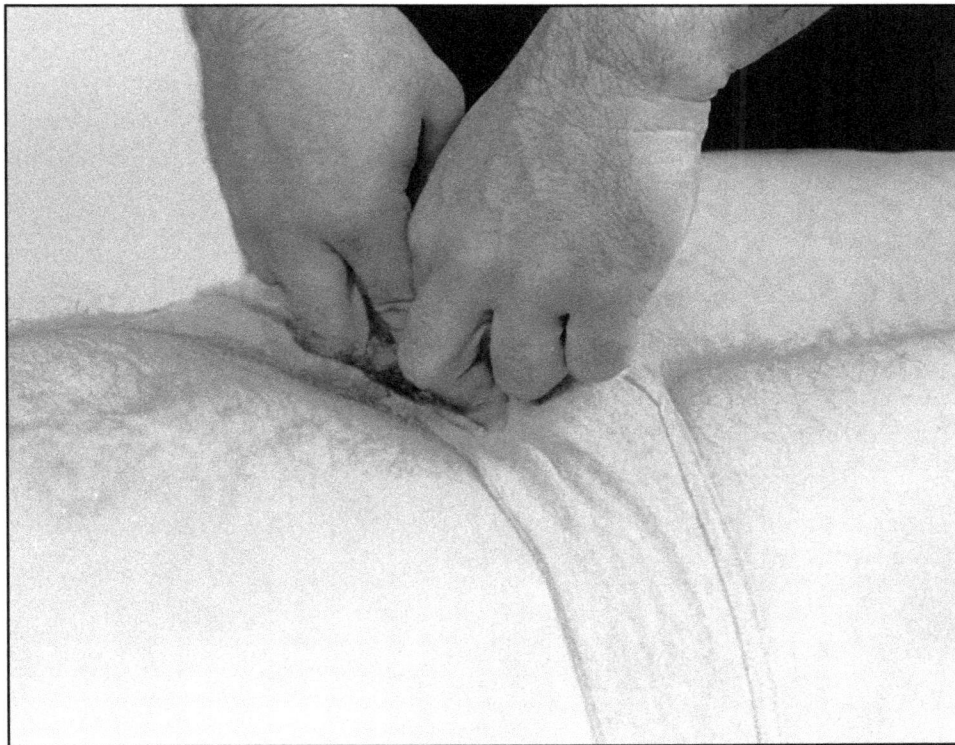

Supine Pelvis Treatment
Pubis Approach

Notes

VENTRAL SACRUM BALANCING

1. Sacro-abdominal Release, Patient Supine Using an Indirect Technique

Fascial attachments between the lumbosacral spine and abdominal visceral structures originate from developmental midline relations. All organs are enveloped in fascia and have ligamentous attachments, inlcuding the tissue remnants of fetal circulation.

Assessment. Operator sits beside the patient with their hand underneath the pelvis on the sacrum, as in a lumbosacral decompression technique. The other hand locates areas in the abdomen which have restriction as determined by areas of hardness, areas of tendeness, etc. Of particular interest are the areas where the remnants of the fetal circulation exist, specifically the urachus and umbilicus. These are areas where myofascial stress is often the greatest. The urachus is located mid line between the umbilicus and the pubes. The palpating hand and the abdomen should come together in a clump over an area of restriction and gently progress downward into the tissue of the belly until a point of maximum restriction is contacted. From here, the tissue should be twisted and side-bent and moved in a manner which reduces this point of tension, creating ease at the point of contact. Movements of the hand on the sacrum can also be used to reduce this tension, bringing the sacrum into flexion or extension, side-bending, and rotation as needed to bring about a sense of relaxation of the area of tension in the abdominal region.

Treatment begins as this tension is reduced, and an unwinding occurs in the palpating abdominal hand as well as in the sacrum. This unwinding will come to a rest and the abdominal tension should be reassessed. Treatment can be similarly carried out over and around the umbilicus or above the pubic bone, depending on where the point of maximum tension is and additionally at visceral contacts within the abdominal cavity.

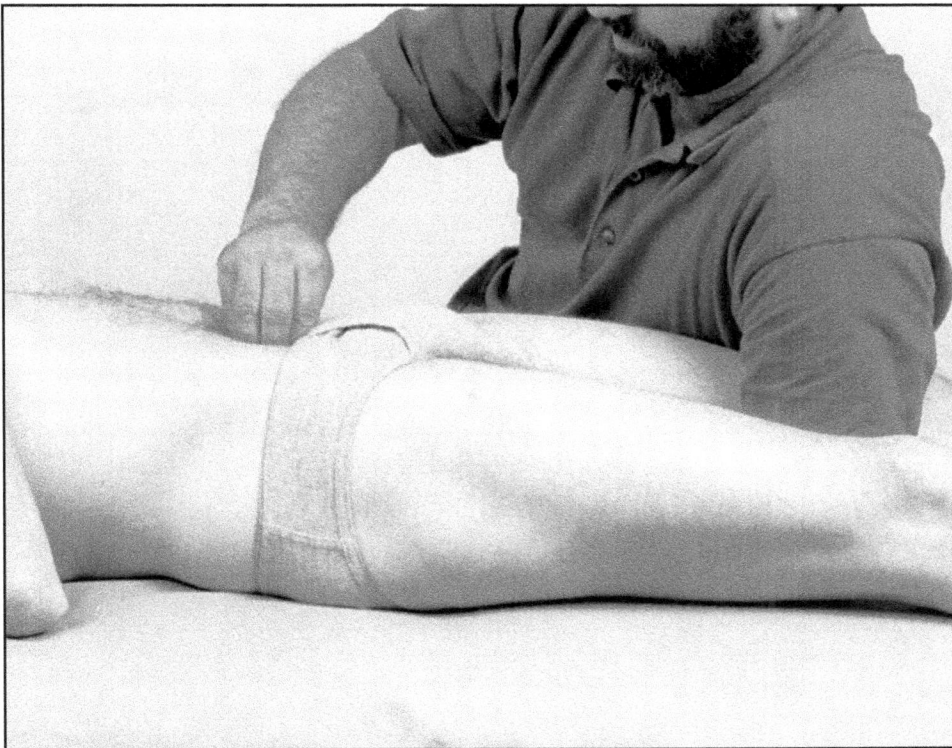

Supine Sacro-Abdominal Treatment

2. Sacrosternal Release, Patient Supine Using a Direct Unwinding Technique

The patient is contacted at the sacrum as before, with the other hand contacting the lower costal cage at the sternal midline. The entire costal cage can be **assessed** with compression, translation left/right, superiorly/inferiorly, rotation and some side-bending to assess compliance and restriction of myofascial tissues. A point of maximal restriction into the barrier should be determined, with the costal cage and the sacrum then moved to a position that increases this sense of tension.

Treatment with myofascial release should occur and an unwinding proceed as in previous techniques. The sacrum can be gently pumped into the sense of the barrier as described in other techniques. This may enhance the release. Sternal compliance should be reassessed at the end of treatment.

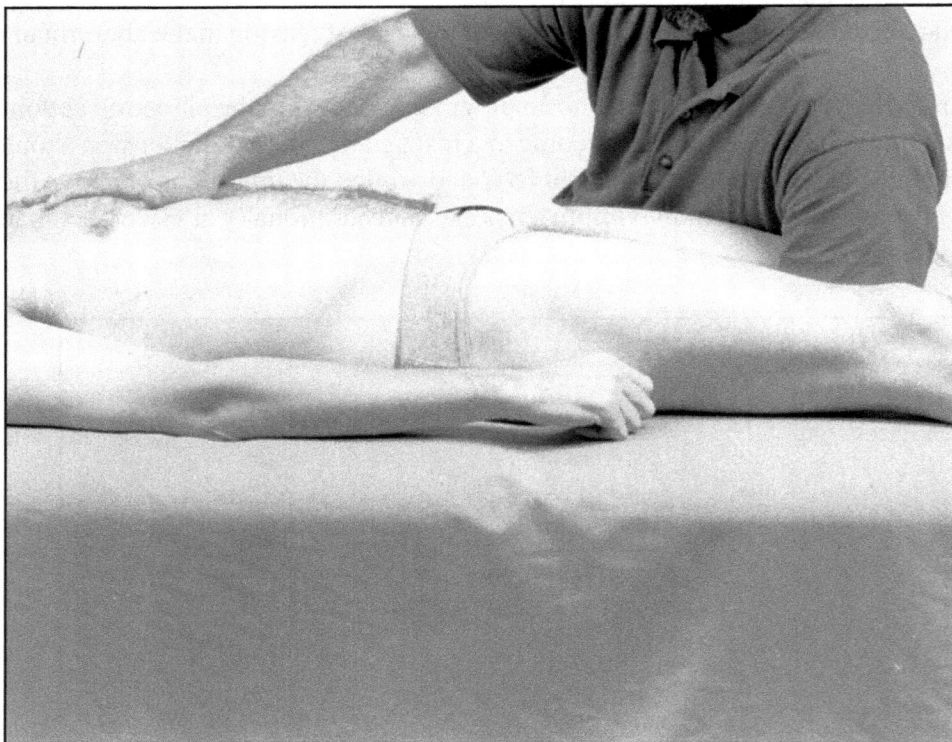

Supine Sacrosternal Treatment

MULTIPLE OPERATOR TECHNIQUES

1. Double Operator Technique, One on the Sacrum and One Using Bilateral Upper Extremities, Patient Supine Using a Direct Unwinding Technique

One operator should sit and put his hand underneath the pelvis on the sacrum, as in previous exercises. The other is standing above the patient's head, contacting both forearms in a fully abducted/flexed position. **Assessment** should include each examiner sensing the tension of his contact area and the tension created by the other operator if they put traction into their respective body contacts. Each operator should test the general area of contact for motion compliance usidng side-bending, rotation, extension, flexion, translation, etc., as described in previous techniques. A point of maximal restriction should be found in each operator's palpatory field and the barrier held until an unwinding occurs. Both operators should **treat** following the unwinding until it comes to rest, at which time both should return and re-assess independently the patient's motion mechanics.

2. Double Operator Technique, One on the Upper Thorax and One on the Bilateral Lower Extremities, Patient Supine Using a Direct Unwinding Technique

One operator sits at the head of the table with both hands underneath the patient's thoracic spine at the paravertebral and costal cage region. The other operator stands at the foot of the patient and contacts both lower extremities posteriorly along the Achilles tendon attachments. Each operator should **assess** independently the motion mechanics at his palpating hand and ask his partner to put gentle traction into his hand contact so as to appreciate the changes that occur when this tension is placed in the myofascial mechanism. For **treatment**, both operators find the point of maximal restriction, using the motion pairs previously described, including traction and compression. Total body unwinding should follow and reassessment performed after treatment.

3. Four Operator Technique, Patient Supine Using an Indirect Technique

In this technique, it is critical that the patient completely relax, so that the movements stimulate a deep sensory motor response in the cortex and cerebellar motor patterning mechanism. This technique will stimulate unwinding of deep coordinated movement patterns from early childhood and infancy. The autonomic nervous system will also respond to this unwinding through central and spinal mechanisms associated with sensory motor programming. In the process of this unwinding it is important to follow each pattern to its "still point" and then wait to see if an additional unwinding movement begins before finishing with treatment. Patients will experience a profound relaxation of various neurophysiological control mechanisms and should take a moment to focus on any changes in normal physiology (e.g. breathing, heart rate, muscle tone, skin color, facial expression.)

Each operator holds onto one of four contact points: the head, the two upper extremities individually, and the two lower extremities simultaneously. Each operator should find his direction of ease with respect to side-bending, rotation, flexion, extension, and then add traction in order to activate the unwinding process. Each operator should follow the slow and progressive unwinding, being careful to avoid the other operators in the process of this total body unwinding. The patient may move around the table, may change from supine to prone, and may even come off of the table in this process. Operators must be certain to support the patient, especially the head, at all times so that the patient may relax throughout this entire process.

<u>Notes</u>

SFIMMS SERIES IN NEUROMUSCULOSKELETAL MEDICINE

MYOFASCIAL AND FASCIAL-LIGAMENTOUS APPROACHES

IN OSTEOPATHIC MANIPULATIVE MEDICINE

Level II

Objectives
Level II

Review concepts from Myofascial Release I, including diagnostic approach, screening exam, and therapeutic process.

Introduce the concept of Release Enhancing Maneuvers

Learn and apply Release Enhancing Maneuvers for cranial nerve facilitation

Introduce the concept of the fulcrum to facilitate diagnostic touch and therapeutic potency

Apply the concept of the fulcrum to treatment of the entire patient.

Explore aspects of craniofascial continuity in the core envelope and its related dural sheaths

Introduce the concept of dynamic fascial-ligamentous release

Apply the concept of dynamic fascial-ligamentous release for the upper and lower extremities

Learn and practice the osteopathic myofascial techniques of William Sutherland, DO

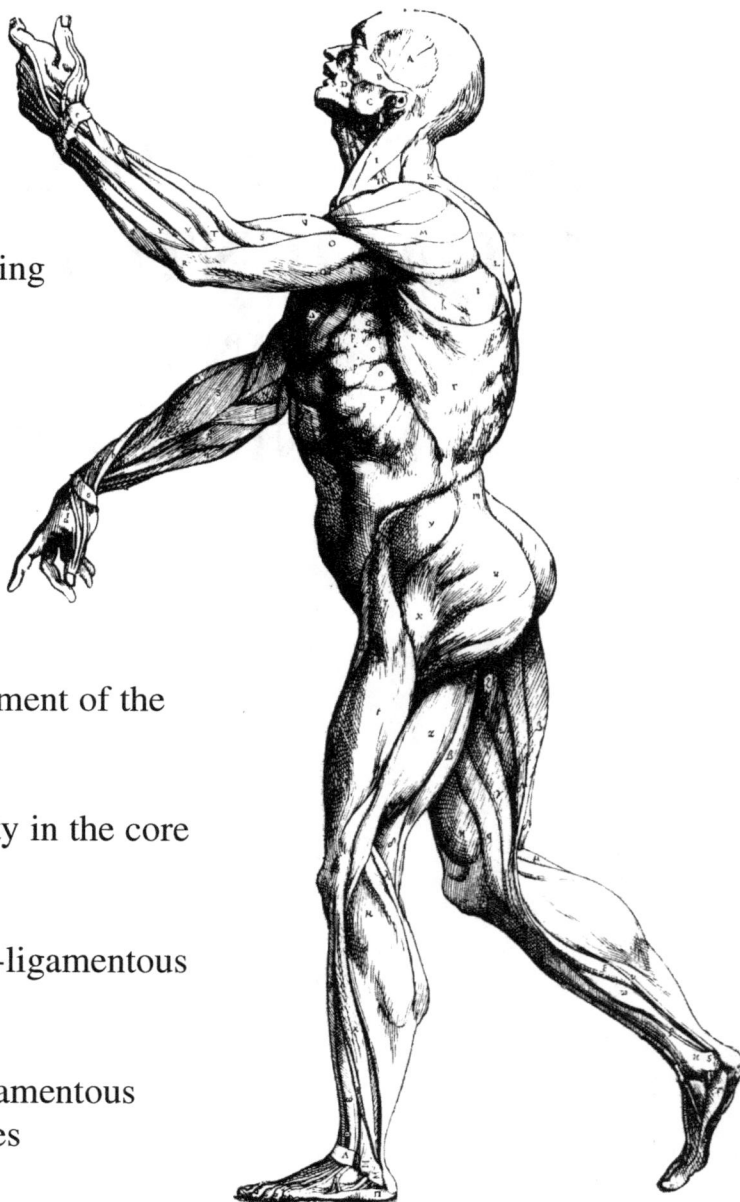

MYOFASCIAL RELEASE CONCEPT

Myofascial and fascial ligamentous release is a manipulative approach that addresses the three-dimensional mobile function/dysfunction of both active (neuroreflexive, neuromuscular properties) and passive (viscoelastic, connective tissue properties) components of the musculoskeletal system.

Three-dimensional layering of myofascial tissue is assessed for relative balance (tightness and looseness) between left and right, front and back, as well as proximal and distal structures.

Treatment with myofascial and fascial ligamentous release uses direct stretching and pumping as well as indirect and direct unwinding techniques to effect neuroreflexive and viscoelastic changes underlying and distant from the point of contact. Three-dimensional perception of anatomic relationships is essential.

Treatment skills require assessment of superficial and deep myofascial tissues for functional balance, i.e., tightness and looseness, as well as sensing viscoelastic and neuroreflexive changes (i.e., creep, hysteresis) under sustained manual loads.

PATIENT ASSESSMENT

Optimal posture is expressed through structural and functional symmetry of static and dynamic activities. Proper co-ordination of all musculoskeletal elements requires proprioception, flexibility, segmental reflexes and muscle balance. Myofascial tension influences all these functions uniquely resulting in relative imbalance, stiffness, immobility and neurologic facilitation.

Myofascial testing procedures assess mobile responses at the initiation of motion and throughout the mobile range. Relative three-dimensional compliance is compared left to right observing the side that encounters resistance first.

Ten-Step Myofascial Screening Exam

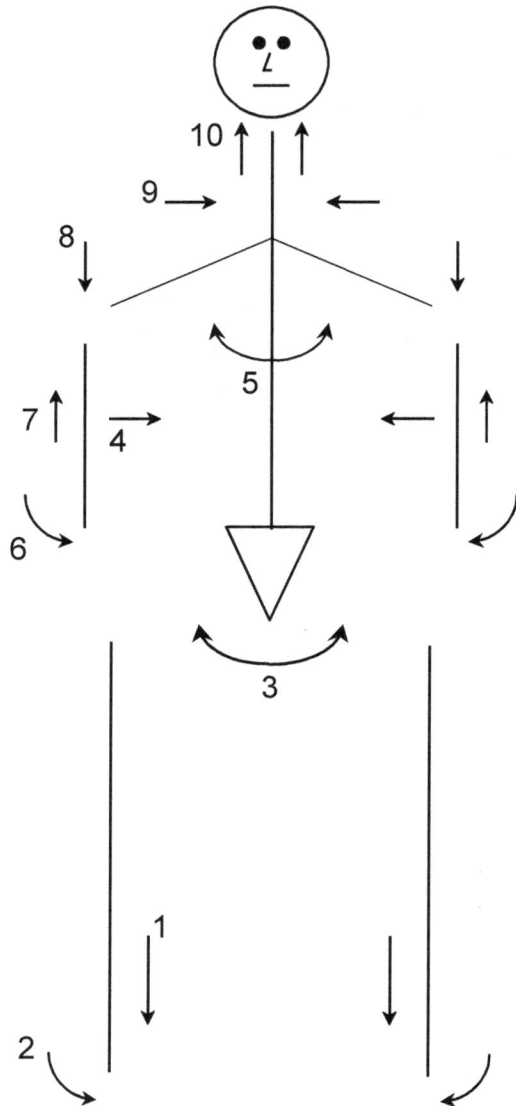

Compare findings for
↑ resistance (↓ compliance) L to R:

1. Traction test
2. Ankle inversion test
3. Pelvic rock
4. Costal cage translation
5. Costal cage compression
6. Forearm pronation
7. Shoulder abduction traction
8. Thoracic rock
9. Lateral cervical compression
10. Occipital traction

PRINCIPLES OF TREATMENT

A. The BBR Concept: Balance, Barrier, Release

1. All body tissues are in a state of balance at the beginning and end of any manual medicine procedure; however, they may be maladapative. Manual medicine procedures deliberately undo this balance in order to reach a more adaptive functional state.

2. Tissue barriers, any impediment to free biomechanical motion, are assessed during manual medicine procedures and are treated by either a direct or indirect approach. As a result, the barrier or tightness should be removed or its influence significantly reduced.

3. At the conclusion of a myofascial or fascial ligamentous release procedure, barriers are released and a deeper sense of tissue balance and inherent motion results. These releases begin to occur at varying time intervals, averaging about 15 to 30 seconds, and are sensed as either a "melting away" of tissue tension or a release of myofascial tightness/ restrictions. Releases may be slow and deliberate or rapid and oscillating reflecting the tissues and body areas being treated.

4. It is frequently true that a number of BBR sequences must occur before myofascial balance is achieved at a level that is associated with clinical functional improvement in the patient's chief complaint. This may also take repeated visits to accomplish.

B. Point of Entry with Tension, Traction, and Twist (POET3)

1. Contacting an area of maximum three-dimensional restriction constitutes a **point of entry** through which the treatment can begin with Myofascial and Fascial Ligamentous Release techniques.

2. The use of **tension** to take up the slack in the tissues and then introducing **traction** and **twist** in either a direct or indirect direction initiates the sequence of Myofascial and Fascial Ligamentous Release.

3. Techniques may use direct stretch along curvilinear planes of myofascial tension (this is where the twist comes in), or pumping techniques wherein the side that is "loose" is compressed to the barrier and the side that is "tight" is gently pumped with a slow compressive rhythmic force. Unwinding techniques use three-dimensional forces, coupling either direct or indirect forces to cause a sustained tissue release or unwinding. This unwinding should be followed until it comes to a point of rest, after which the tissues should be reassessed for three-dimensional symmetry. If asymmetry persists, the procedure should be repeated until tissue balance is improved.

C. Proximal and Distal Releases

1. It is important that the operator is focused and relaxed in order to enhance the ability to perceive and follow changes in the myofascial tissue. This requires a receptive mind and palpatory sense with which to follow inherent releases that are occuring underneath their hands. This is distinct fom "pushing tissues around" in the direction they should go or should be in. Any given Myofascial or Fascial Ligamentous Release may involve tissues at both a proximal and distal source, which makes release a unique and potentially far-reaching manual medicine procedure. Sensing tissue restrictions and releases along myofascial planes to distal regions of the body can be developed through visualizing total body anatomy and projecting palpatory awareness.

RELEASE-ENHANCING MANEUVERS FOR MYOFASCIAL AND INTEGRATED NEUROMUSCULAR RELEASE

Based on osteopathic approaches developed by Dr. Robert C. Ward, D.O.

Myofascial techniques focus on a point of entry (POET$_3$), using tension, traction, and twist. Active and passive mechanisms are engaged in this process. Distal mechanical and reflex responses are often noted, and are related to larger integrative aspects of sensory, motor, autonomic, supraspinal, and visceral functions. In order to facilitate these responses, the patient may be instructed to perform a motor behavior which further engages active and passive mechanisms, (i.e., increase or decrease palpatory tensions perceived by the operator). Such release-enhancing maneuvers (REM's) may involve simple head rotation, arm extension, respiratory cooperation, eye movements, and even memory retrieval.

Table Session: Take an area of maximal body tension and mobile restriction from the screening exam findings. Focusing bilateral hand contact on this point of entry, local tension, traction and twist are applied while simultaneously requesting the patient to actively engage release enhancing maneuvers. These REMs should be extrapolated from other significant findings noted in the screening exam. (i.e. shoulder abduction, forearm pronation, head rotation and/or sidebending, thoracic cage side bending, hip flexion/extension, ankle eversion/ inversion or dorsi/plantarflexion) Multiple REMs should be introduced and responses noted at the point of local contact. Responses may increase tension or balance tensions palpated locally by the operator, in either case, local forces applied by the operator can be direct or indirect. In this way releases can be deeper and more systemic facilitating a more integrated and sustained tissue and motor system response. Treatment can be carried out supine or prone and with multiple operators if desired.

Cranial Nerve and Proprioceptive Facilitation

A subset of release enhancing maneuvers have focused on cranial nerve facilitation of myofascial and integrated neuromuscular releases. Sensorimotor linkages are controlled in five brain centers; the spinal cord, the brain stem, the cerebral cortex, the cerebellum, and the basal ganglia. Anatomic and functional continuity of cranial nerve function has been observed and is evident in such mechanisms as vision compensating for proprioceptive deficits. Linkages can also be observed in visual and auditory stimulation of reflex motor responses, i.e., bright lights or loud noises. Visual, olfactory, and digestive functions have obvious linkages.

Motor function is reflexively modulated by pain and mechanical dysfunction through inhibition and excitation, centrally and peripherally. Central pathways in particular have functional and structural associations with cranial nerve outflow and feedback mechanisms. This produces coordination deficits in cranial nerve activities as well as postural reflexes and system-wide proprioceptive function

Specific cranial nerve and proprioceptive release-enhancing maneuvers have been shown to be quite productive in patients with chronic head, craniocervical, cervicothoracic, and upper extremity syndromes. These patients often demonstrate faulty proprioceptive and asymmetric cranial nerve motor function. Common problem areas include the mouth, tongue, oral pharynx, jaw, face, eyes, and voice. Asymmetrical responses to these motor functions can be observed in craniocervical, cervicothoracic, shoulder, and upper limb functions. Release-enhancing maneuvers can be applied to other body regions with success, especially when palpatory findings direct the operator to clinically significant regions of the body demonstrating dysfunction.

Cranial Nerve and Proprioceptive Facilitation: Assessment and Treatment

Assessment:

The following protocol has been developed to assess in particular cranial nerve facilitation. The patient is examined in a standing position for increased and asymmetrical <u>resting tone</u> of the suboccipital and cervicothoracic junctions. The remaining assessments are all carried out while contacting the suboccipital or cervicothoracic junction, whichever has the greatest resting tone. Postural reflexes are noted in these areas while the patient assumes <u>one-legged standing maneuvers</u>, comparing the response to performance of this maneuver between the left and right lower limbs. Asymmetrical responses may also be noted on the left or right side of the patient's body. The patient is then instructed to assume a supine position while the following cranial nerve facilitations are carried out (demonstrations of these techniques are shown on the following pages):

(1) **Eye movements**, including cranial nerves three, four, and six. Horizontal gaze left and right, vertical gaze superior and inferior, oblique gaze left superior, left inferior, right superior, right inferior.

(2) **Jaw thrust**, cranial nerve number five. Thrust left, thrust right, bilateral thrust (protrusion) and bilateral retrusion.

(3) **Facial muscles**, cranial nerve number seven. Smile, frown, surprise.

(4) **Throat muscles**, cranial nerve number nine. Swallowing.

(5) **Vocalization**, Cranial nerve number ten.

(6) **Shoulder shrug**, cranial nerve number eleven.

(7) **Tongue thrust**, cranial nerve number twelve. Thrust left, thrust right.

Responses to these maneuvers are noted to all generally increase tension in the suboccipital or cervicothoracic junction region being tested. A grading system should be used to assess the amount of increased tension occurring at these areas (+++, ++, +), as well as any asymmetry in the increased tension between the left- and right-sided responses. Modulation can be observed by slight variations in motor performance. Modulators include left or right sided eyebrow raising, high vs. low notes with vocalization, left or right sided shoulder shrug, etc.

Treatment:

•Significant increases in tension and/or asymmetry are noted, and the patient is instructed to apply these behaviors as release-enhancing maneuvers in carrying out myofascial and integrative neuromuscular releases. Behaviors should be combined for more effective responses, and can be combined with other REMs including one-legged standing. After treatment, one-legged standing should be repeated to assess changes in proprioceptive and postrual reflexes.

•Patients are then instructed to perform combinations of these motor activities at home for continued rehabilitative efforts in enhancing coordinated motor function.

Cranial Nerves and
Craniofacial and Cervical Muscle Innervations

CN I	Olfactory	Sensory	
CN II	Optic	Sensory	
CN III	Oculomotor	Motor	Superior rectus Medial rectus Inferior rectus Inferor oblique Levator palpebrae superioris
CN IV	Trochlear	Motor	Superior oblique
CN V	Trigeminal Mandibular branch	Motor/ Sensory	Masseter Temporalis Anterior digastric Mylohyoid Tensor tympani Tensor veli palatini
CN VI	Abducens	Motor	Lateral rectus
CN VII	Facial	Motor/ Sensory	Posterior digastric Occipitalis Frontalis Buccinator Posterior auricular Facial expression Stylohyoid Stapedius
CN VIII	Vestibulocochlear	Sensory	Affects proprioception and cerebellar functions
CN IX	Glossopharyngeal	Motor/ Sensory	Stylopharyngeus Pharyngeal constrictors (with X & XI)
CN X	Vagus	Motor/ Sensory	Larynx Pharyngeal constrictors (with IX & XI) Palatoglossus
CN XI	Accessory	Motor	Pharyngeal constrictors (with IX & X) Sternocleidomastoid Trapezius
CN XII	Hypoglossal	Motor	Tongue intrinsics Genioglossus Hyoglossus Styloglossus
C1,2,3	Ansa cervicalis		Infrahyoid group
C1-8			Scalenes
C4,5	Dorsal scapular		Rhomboids Levator scapulae
C 6,7,8	Thoracodorsal		Latissiumus dorsi
C5,6,7,8,T1	Lateral and Medial Pectoral		Pectoralis major and minor

Cranial Nerve Facilitation

		Subocciput	CT jxn	Modulation
Resting tone				
One-leg stand	L			
	R			
Eyes (III, IV, VI)				
Horizontal Gaze	L			
	R			
Vertical Gaze	S			
	I			
Oblique Gaze	LS			
	LI			
	RS			
	RI			
Jaw (V)				
Thrust	L			
	R			
	Bi			
Retrusion	Bi			
Face (VII)				
Smile				
Frown				
Surprise				
Throat (IX)				
Swallow				
Vocalization (X)				
Shoulder Shrug (XI)				
Tongue (XII)				
Thrust	L			
	R			

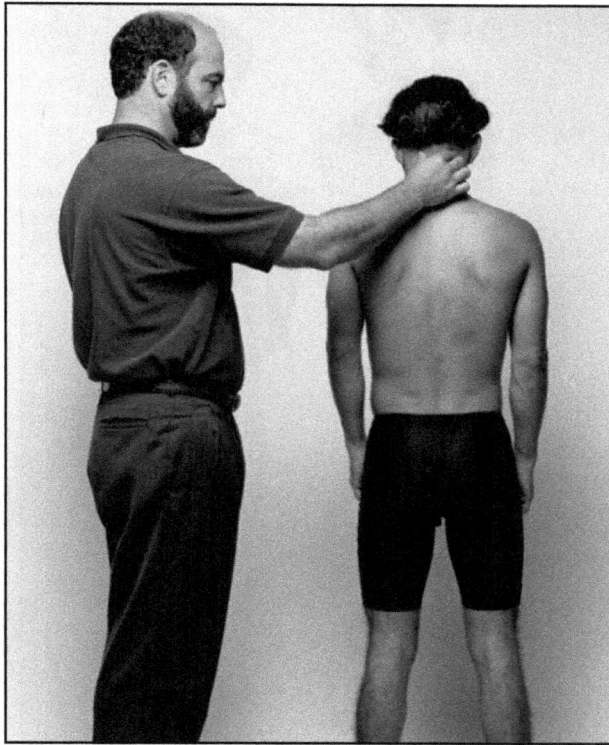

Testing for Suboccipital Resting Tone

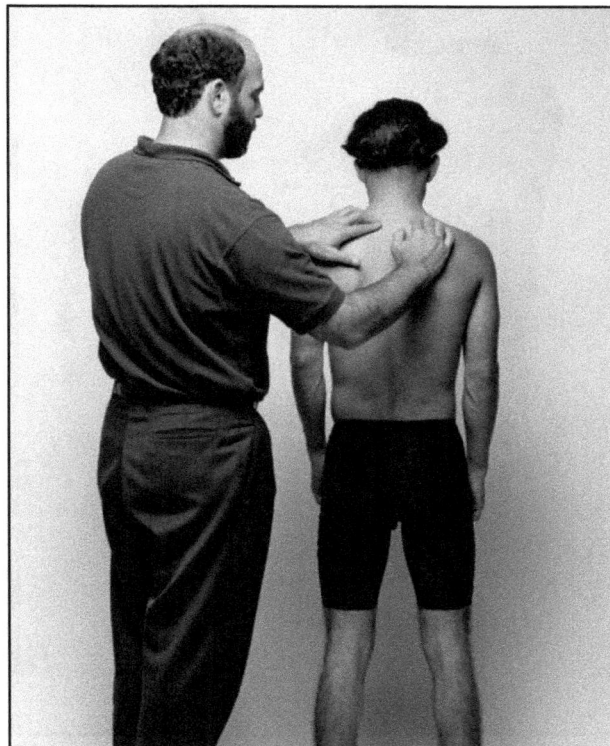

Testing Resting Tone of the Cervicalthoracic Junction

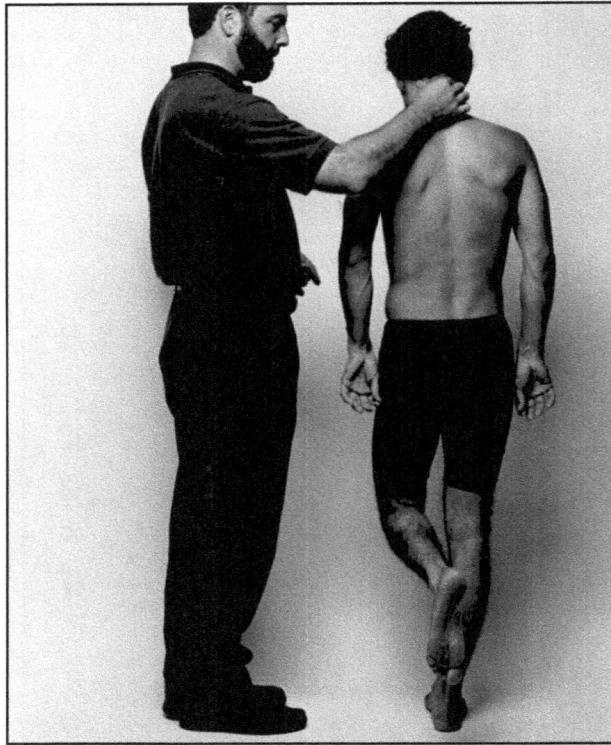

Testing Postural Reflexes of the Suboccipital Area During
One-Legged Standing Maneuver

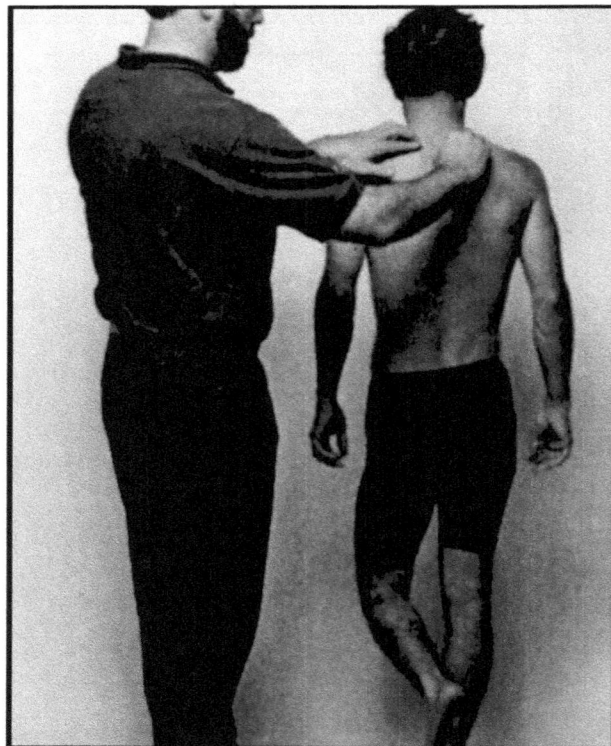

Testing Postural Reflexes of the Cervicothoracic Junction
During One-Legged Standing Maneuver

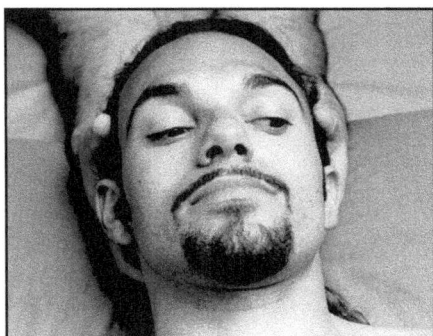

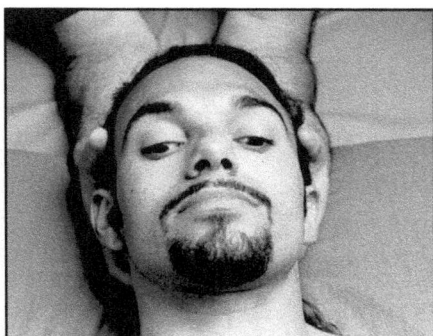

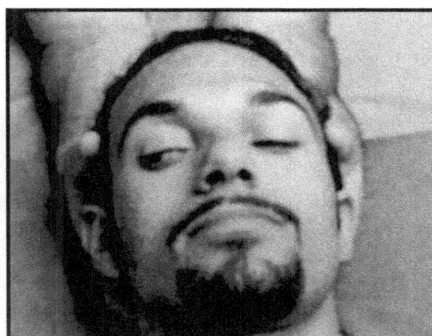

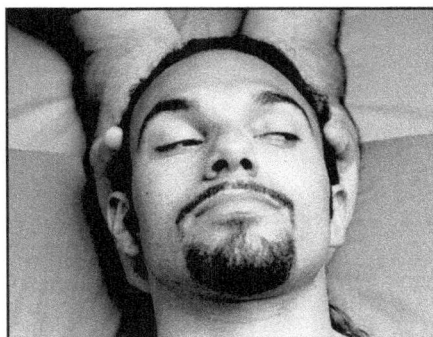

Eye Movements

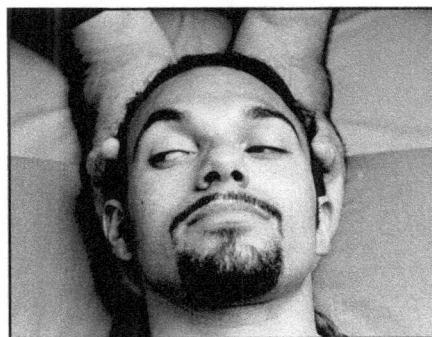

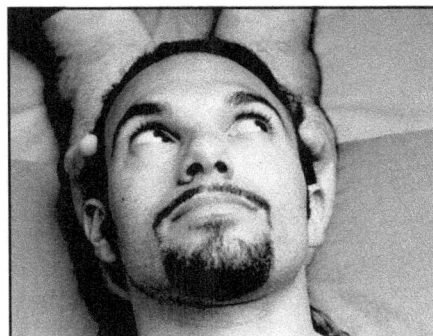

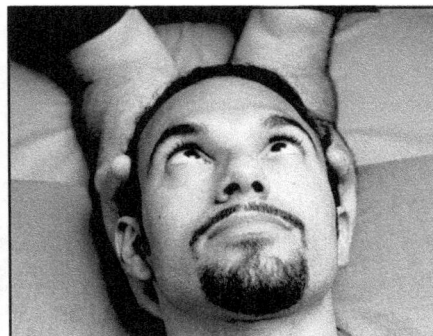

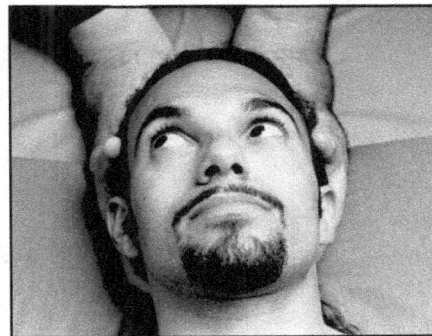

Testing Eye movements. Clockwise from Middle Top: Vertical Inferior, Oblique Right Inferior, Horizontal Right, Oblique Right Superior, Vertical Superior, Oblique Left Superior, Horizontal Left, Oblique Left Inferior.

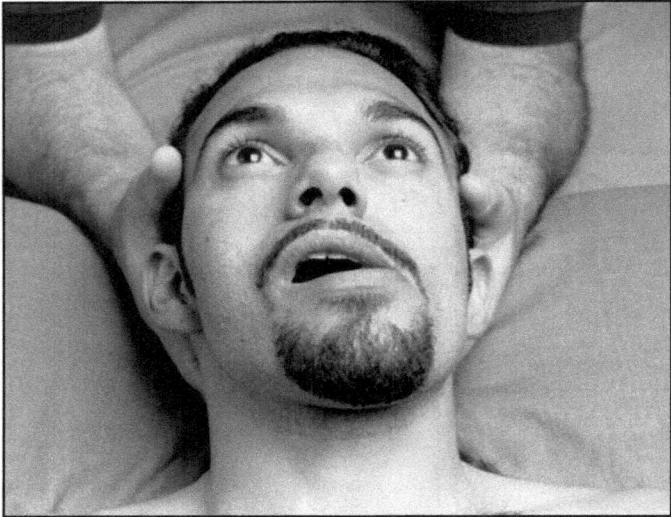

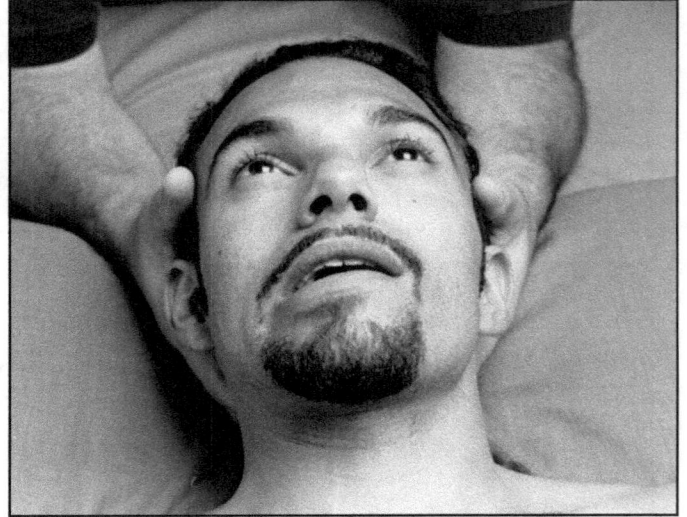

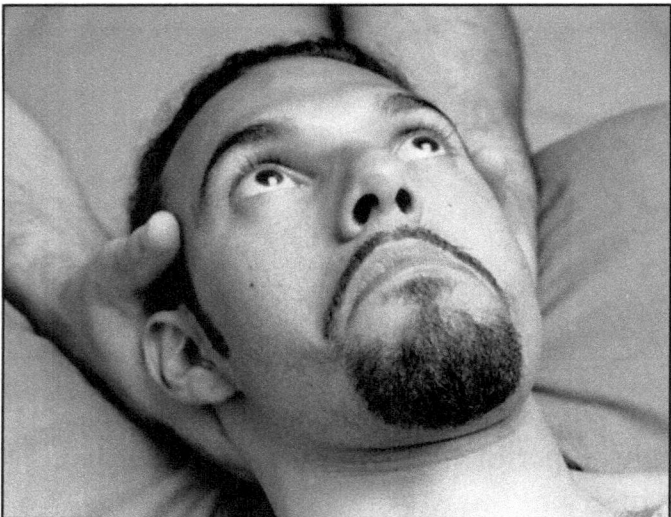

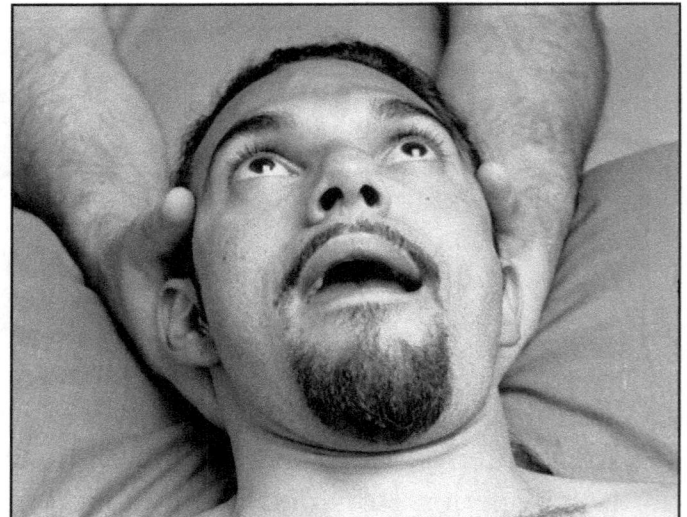

Jaw Thrusts. Clockwise from top left: Thrust Left, Thrust Right, Bilateral Retrusion, Bilateral Protrusion

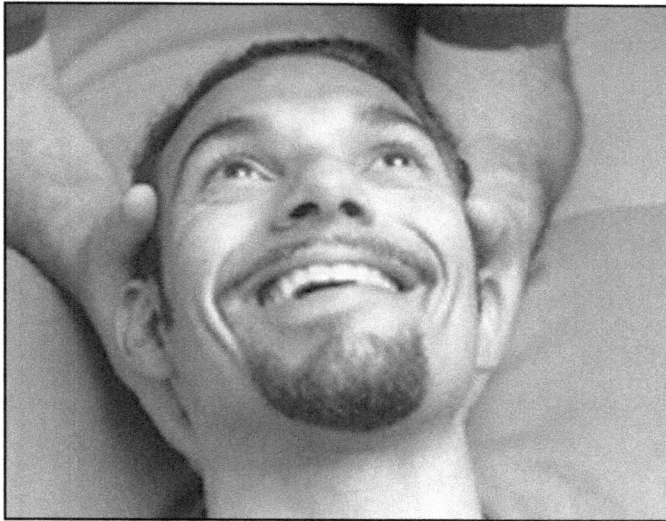

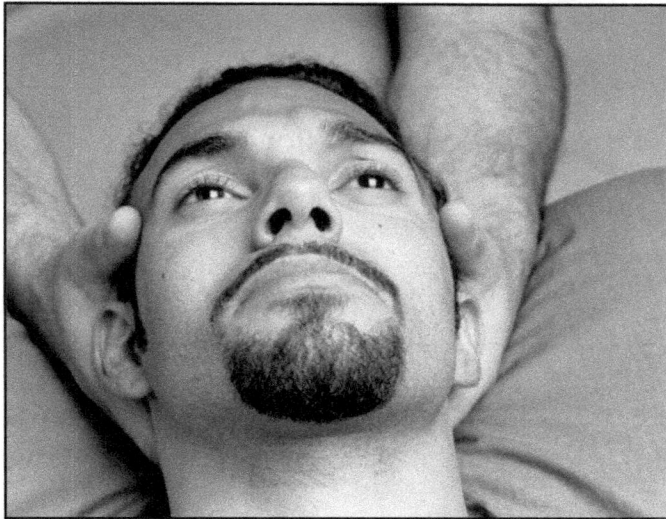

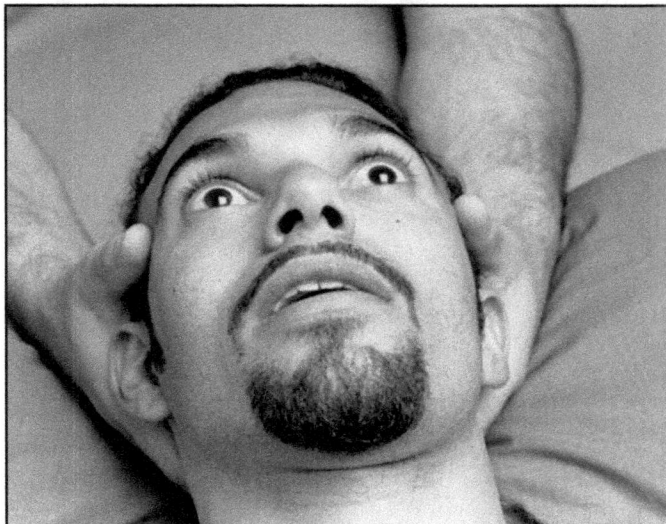

Facial Muscles. From Top: Smile, Frown, Surprise.

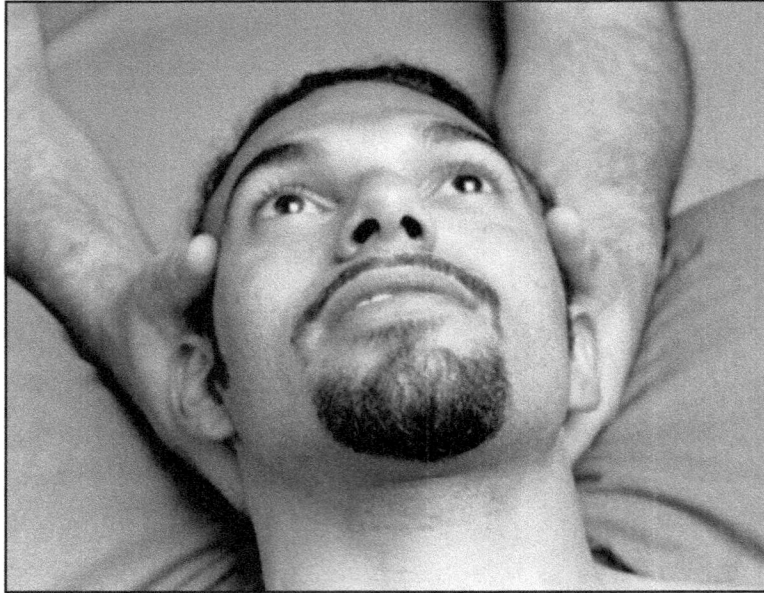

Throat Muscles. Swallowing.

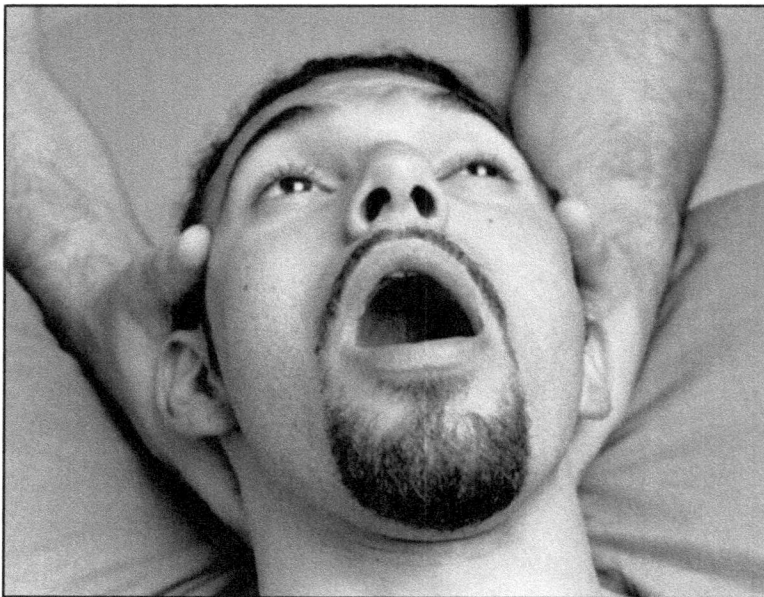

Vocalization

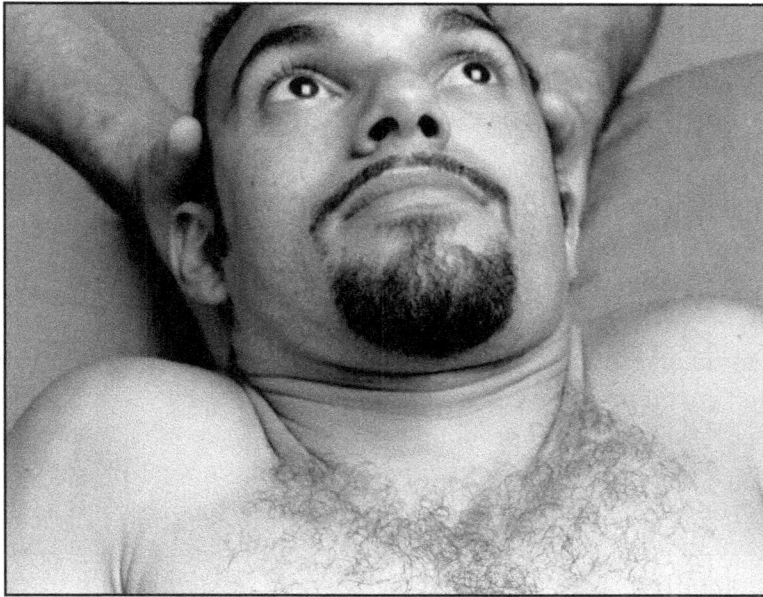

Shoulder Shrug

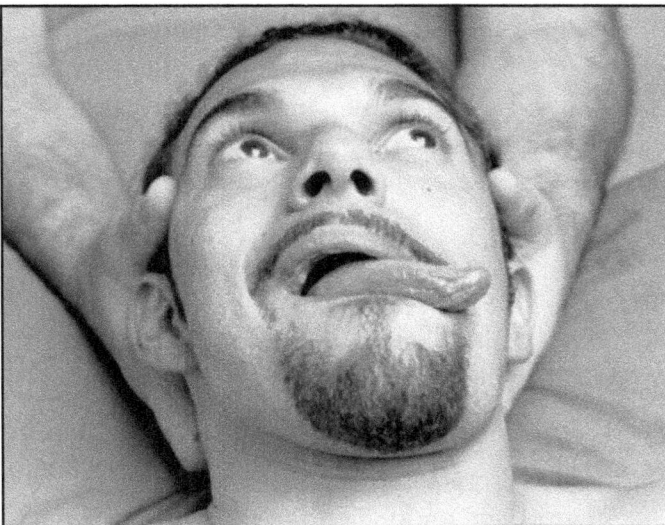

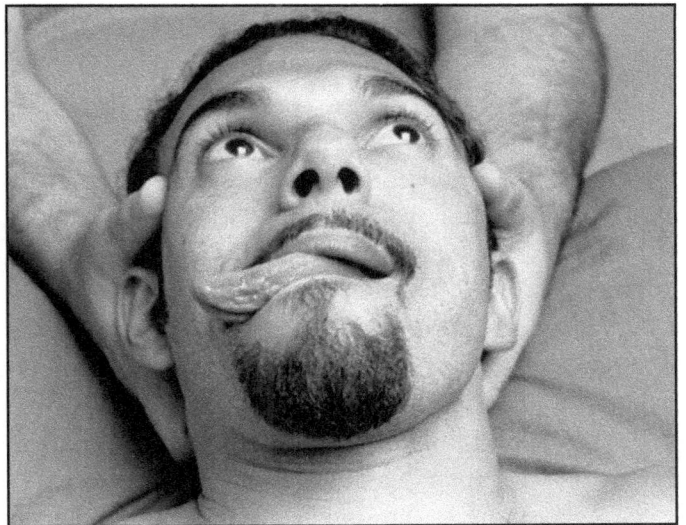

Tongue Thrusts. Thrust Left, Thrust Right.

THE FULCRUM AND DIAGNOSTIC TOUCH

Based on osteopathic approaches developed by Dr. Rollin Becker, DO

I.   The Fulcrum

A.   General Considerations

Diagnosis as an art is an important component in the field of diagnosis. There are three aspects to an encounter between a physician and a patient: The patient's ideas and beliefs of what he/she considers the problem to be; the physician's concept of what he/she considers the problem to be; and that which the anatomical-physiological wholeness of the patient's body knows the problem to be. With respect to the last of these aspects, osteopathic manipulative treatment must allow the physiological function within the patient to manifest its own unerring potency rather than use blind external force. This is accomplished through the use of a dynamic fulcrum, which is the support or point of support on which the lever arm turns in raising or moving something. The dynamic fulcrum itself moves as the forces within the patient respond to therapeutic potency.

The establishment of an appropriate fulcrum facilitates diagnostic touch: the placing of the hands and fingers on the tissues under examination is done with the idea that the fingers can mold themselves to the patient's body. Compression is applied into an area of tissue tension or reduced mobility, and then waiting for the response of the tissues, which will always follow. The establishment of a fulcrum allows the operator to harness the inherent forces within the tissues. The operator listens to and follows the inherent movements of these forces to their physiologic point of balance (neutral point). Neutral point is a point of balanced tension around which dynamic motion within the tissues is functionally organized. A point of balance of this type facilitates the inherent therapeutic potency within the patient and acts as a doorway for this unerring potency to restore tissue symmetry and midline balance.

In summary, there are two tissue unwindings occurring when applying the fulcrum to diagnostic touch. One is the movement of the tissues to reach their point of balanced tension, where the operator forces from the outside match and balance the patient forces on the inside. The second is the expression of the therapeutic potency, which causes an expansive quality to enter the tissues, and is sometimes associated with another unwinding as the tissues are reorganizing around the physiologic midline. It is not an insignificant factor that the operator's therapeutic potency helps to facilitate the expression of the patient's inherent restorative capacity. Essentially, corrective forces are not the result of the application of technique, but rather a cooperative interplay performed in the language of palpatory expression. This enhances the dynamic therapeutic potency present in the perceptual interaction between patient and physician. The operator must be so quiet as to render silent his own presence. This way, he can not only observe the patient's tissue response, but also disappear into the perceptual potency alive in the therapeutic process.

Treatment Sequence:

B. Lower Half of the Body

Patient is supine, the knees are flexed, and the feet placed flat on the table. Lateralization of the feet helps to stabilize the pelvis. Operator sits at the patient's side.

1. Pelvis

One hand molds with the sacrum without wrist deviation. The fingertips of this hand are placed at the level of the spinous process of the fifth lumbar segment (L5). The other arm and hand bridge the anterior superior iliac spine (ASIS) on each side of the pelvis. The elbow that is leaning on the treatment table establishes the fulcrum.

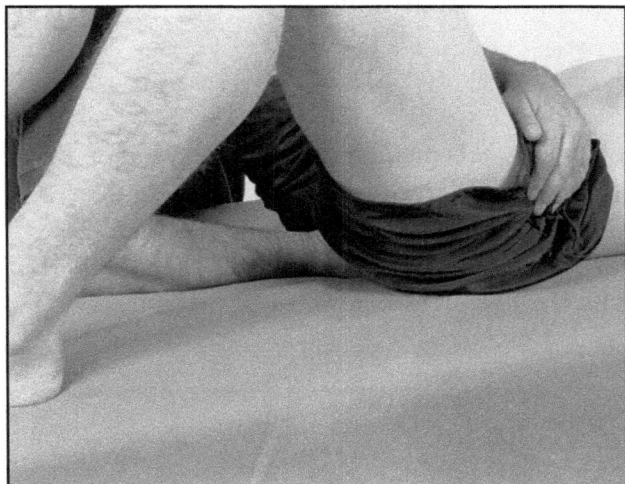

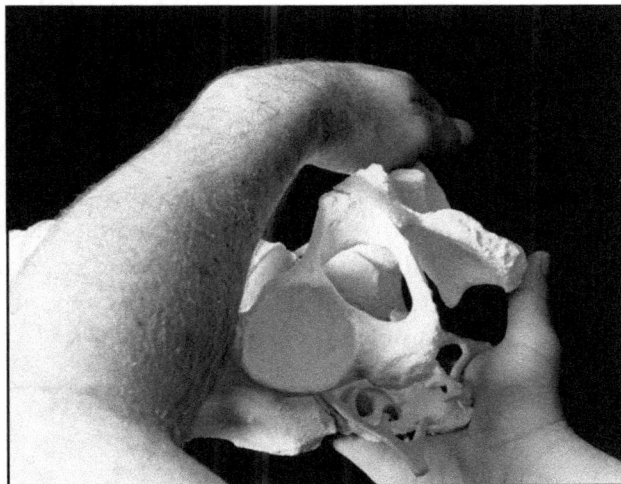

Pelvic Treatment

2. Ilio-Sacrum/Lower Lumbar

One hand molds with the sacrum. The other hand is placed under the iliosacral articulation at a point of perceived tension. The fingertips of this hand may also contact the spinous processes of the lower lumbar segments (L3, 4, 5). The fulcrum is established by both elbows: one leaning on the treatment table (Sacrum), and the other leaning on the table or the physician's knee (Ilio-Sacrum; Lower Lumbar).

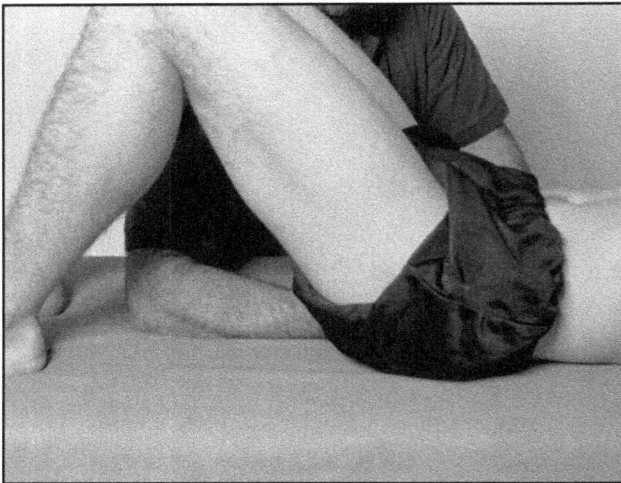

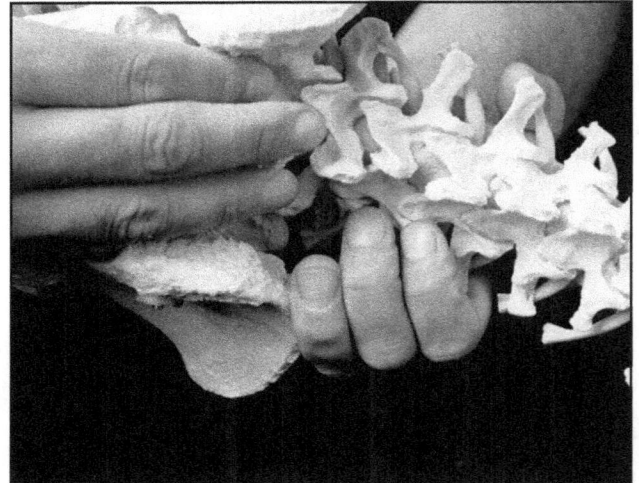

Ilio-Sacrum/Lower Lumbar Treatment

3. Iliacus

One hand molds with the sacrum, the other contacts an area of iliacus tension on the inner shelf of the ilium medial to the ASIS. The fulcrum is established by both elbows, one on the table and the other in the air. Movements into the iliacus muscle follow in directions of ease in conjunction with the respiratory phase (i.e. exhalation). Discomfort may be experienced by the patient so care must be taken to go slowly and gently.

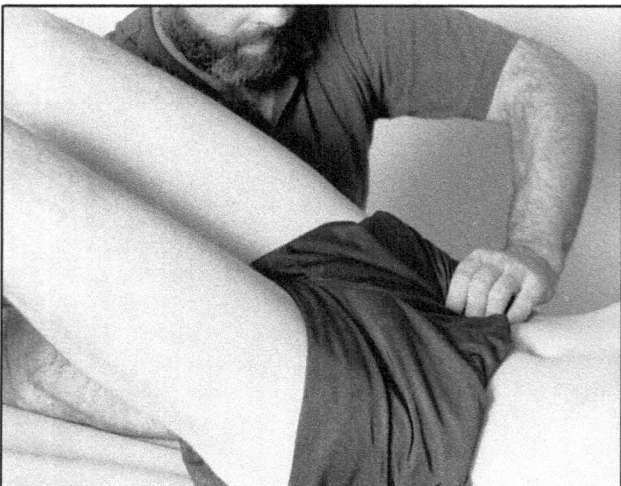

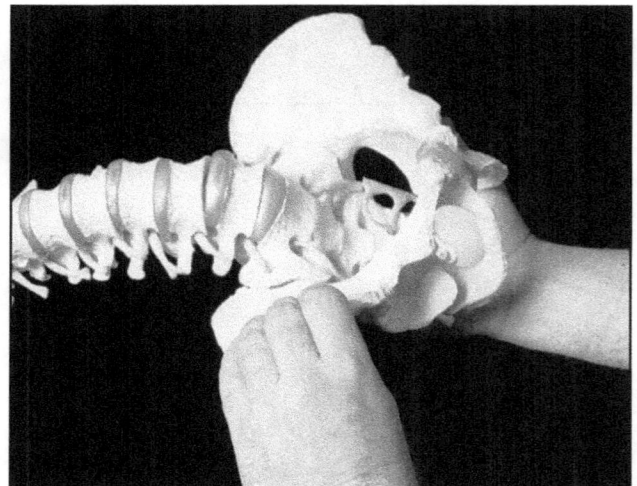

Treatment of Iliacus

4. Abdominal Fascia

One hand molds with the sacrum. The other hand accomplishes multiple assessments: the abdominal quadrants, costal margins, linea alba, tension of the inguinal ligaments, and shear dysfunctions at the pubic symphysis. The fulcrum is established by both elbows: one leaning on the treatment table (Sacrum), and the other being the elbow of the exploring arm (Abdomen).

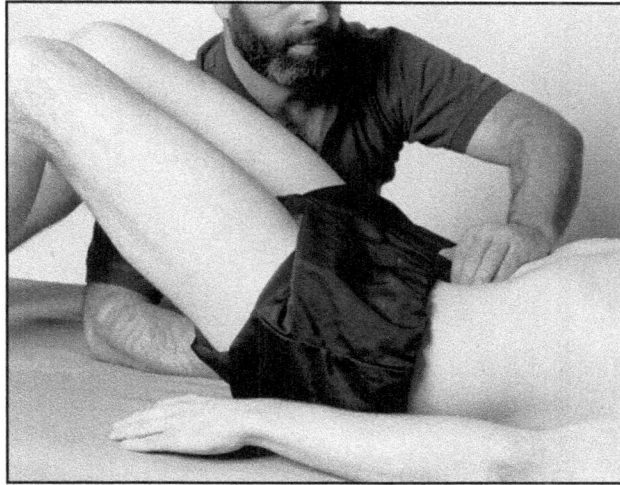

Treatment of Abdominal Fascia

5. Upper Lumbar; Relation to Psoas Muscle and Sacropelvis

One hand is placed under the upper lumbar area. The other arm and hand bridge the flexed knees. The fulcrum is established by the elbow on the operator's knee or table. (Upper Lumbar Area).

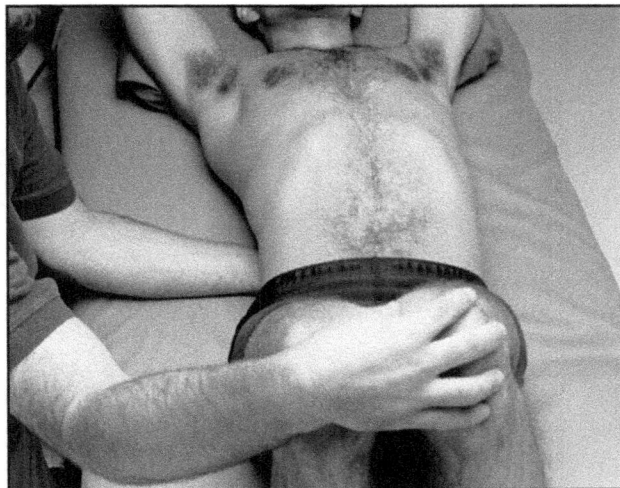

Upper Lumbar Treatment

6. <u>Liver</u>

One hand is placed under the lower ribs beneath the liver. The other hand is placed over the anterior surface of the liver. The fulcrum is established by the elbow on the operator's knee , or on the table in contact with the posterior aspect of the lower ribs.

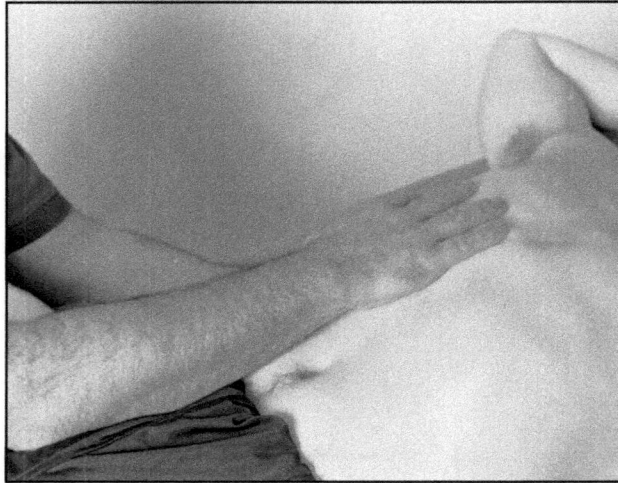

Liver Treatment

7. <u>Sacrosternal Axis</u>

One hand is placed on the sacrum with the patient's hips flexed. The other hand is placed on the midline of the sternum. This is the culmination of the lower sequence, and allows these two important midline structures to come into optimal balance

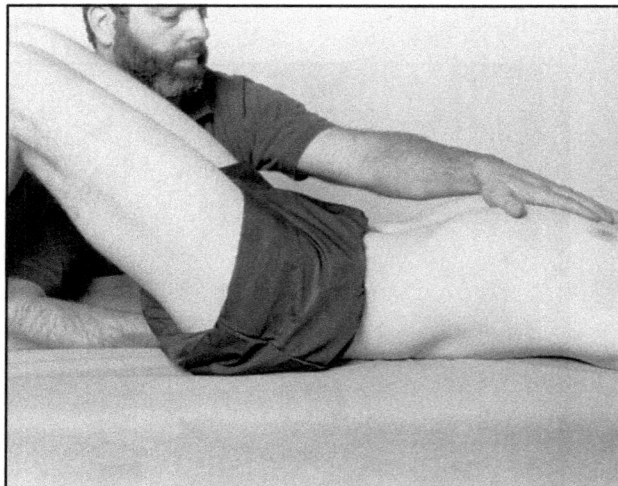

Sacrosternal Axis Treatment

Treatment Sequence:

C. Upper Half of the Body

The patient remains in the position established at the beginning of this evaluation sequence. Operator sits at the head of the table unless indicated otherwise (see 1. Rib Cage).

1. <u>Rib Cage</u>

Operator sits at patient's side. One hand is placed beneath the rib cage at a point of perceived tension, with the fingertips on the transverse processes of the associated thoracic vertebrae. The other hand is placed on the anterior ends of the ribs. The fulcrum is established by the elbow on the knee or table.

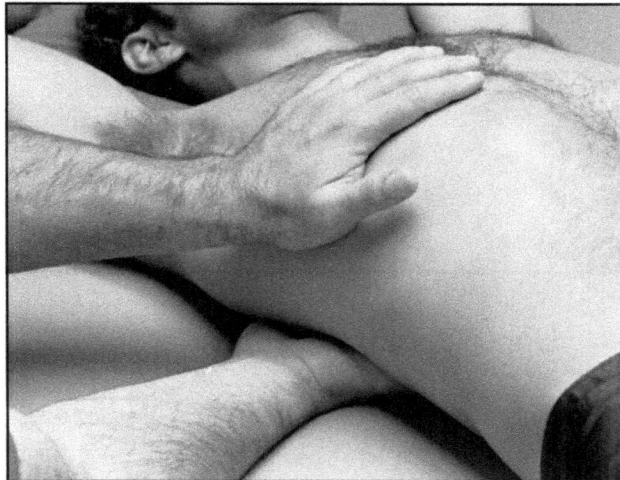

Rib Cage Treatment

2. <u>Lower Thorax</u>

Both hands are placed beneath the patient at the level of the twelfth thoracic segment (T12). This area corresponds to the level of the insertion of the trapezius muscles bilaterally. The fulcrum is established bilaterally by the elbows resting on the tabletop. This procedure can be applied to areas higher in the thoracic cage as well.

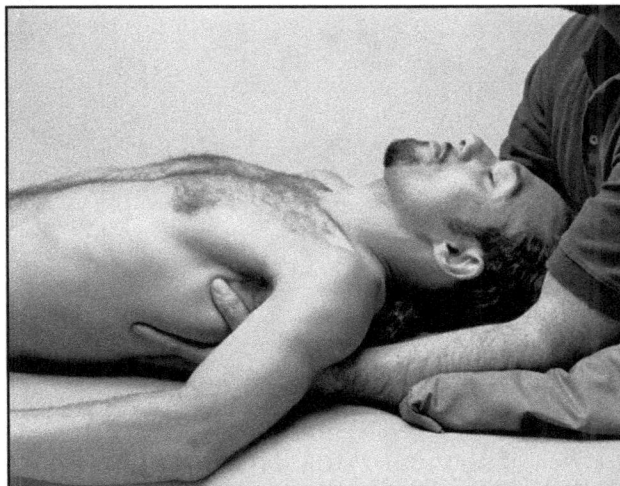

Lower Thorax Treatment

3. **Upper Thorax**

The patient's head rests on a pillow. One hand and arm contact the upper thoracic spinous processes, with the fingers spread slightly to contact the ribs on each side. The opposite hand is placed on the sternum. The fulcrum is established by the elbow on the tabletop, beside the patient's head.

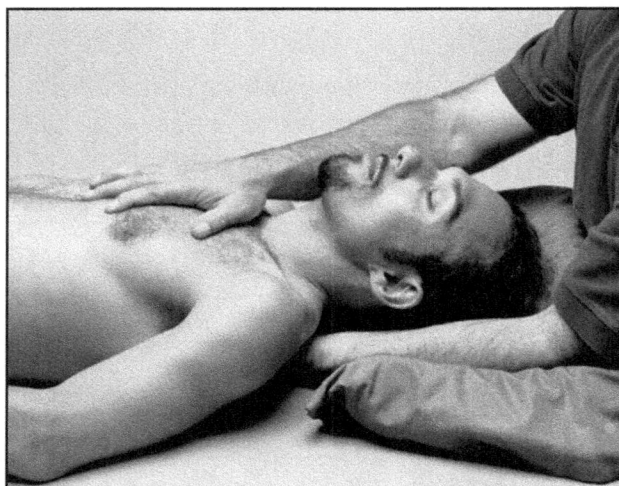

Upper Thorax Treatment

4. **Cervical Area**

Both hands bridge the entire cervical area from the base of the skull to the upper thorax compressing into the lateral tissues. The fulcrum is established bilaterally by the elbows and forearms resting on the tabletop.

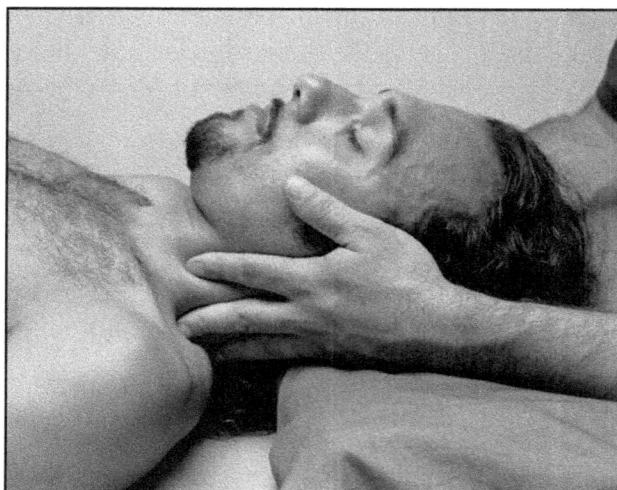

Cervical Area Treatment

5. Cranium and Craniocervical Junction

a. Occipitoatlantal Articulation

One hand contacts the posterior tubercle of the atlas. The opposite hand contacts the vertex of the patient's head. The fulcrum is established by the placement of the elbow on the tabletop. Balanced tension will be perceived at the occipitoatlantal contact as the compressive forces are balanced through the head.

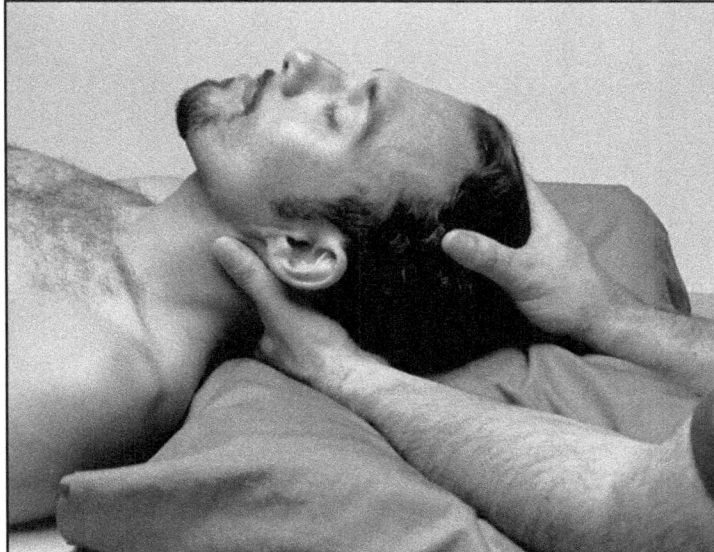

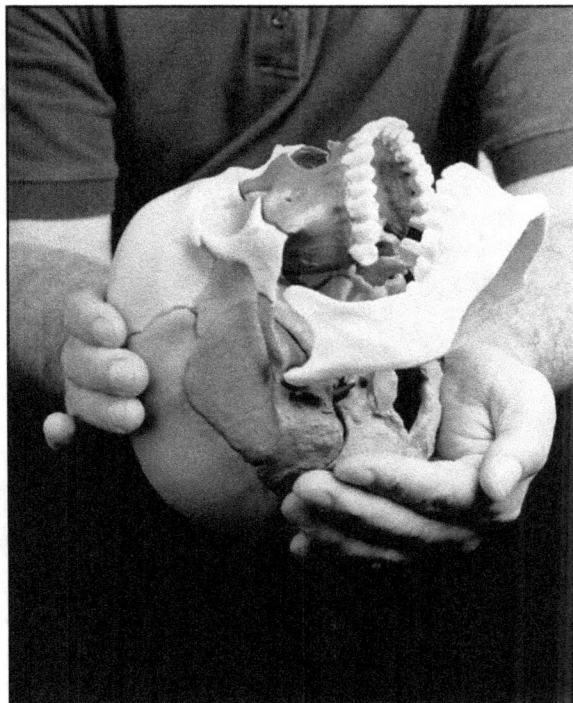

Occipitoatlantal Articulation Treatment

b. <u>Posterior Fossa</u>

The patient's head rests on the interlaced or overlapped fingers of the physician. The physician's thumbs extend above the ears toward the forepart of the head, tracing the course of the tentorium cerebelli. The fulcrum is established by the placement of the elbows on the tabletop.

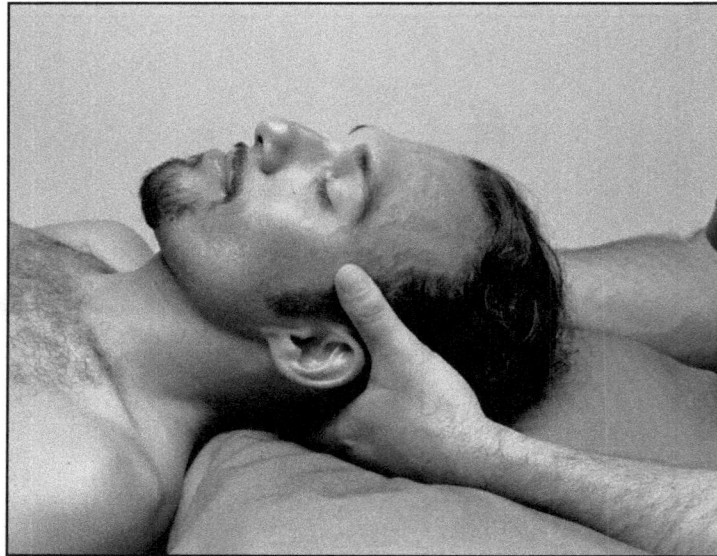

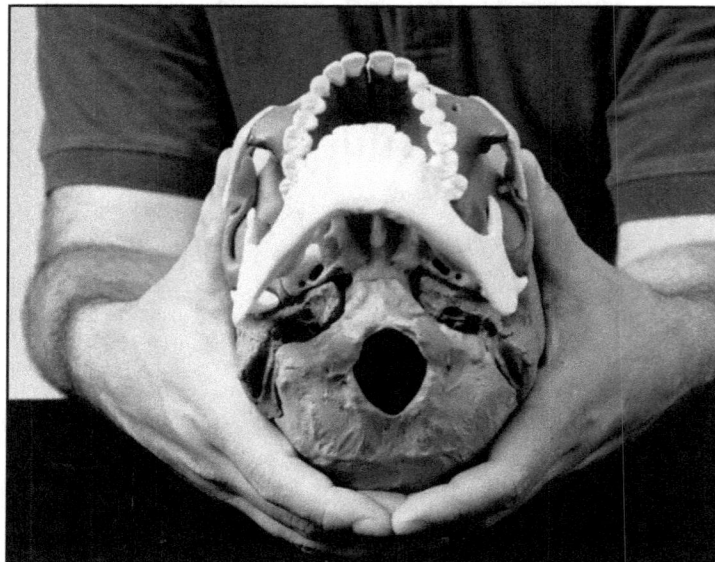

Posterior Fossa Treatment

6. __Occipitosternal Axis__

One hand contacts the midline of the occiput, the other the midline of the sternum. The fulcrum is established by the operator's forearm contact with the table. These being important midline structures, the occiput and the sternum should come into a more optimal midline relation.

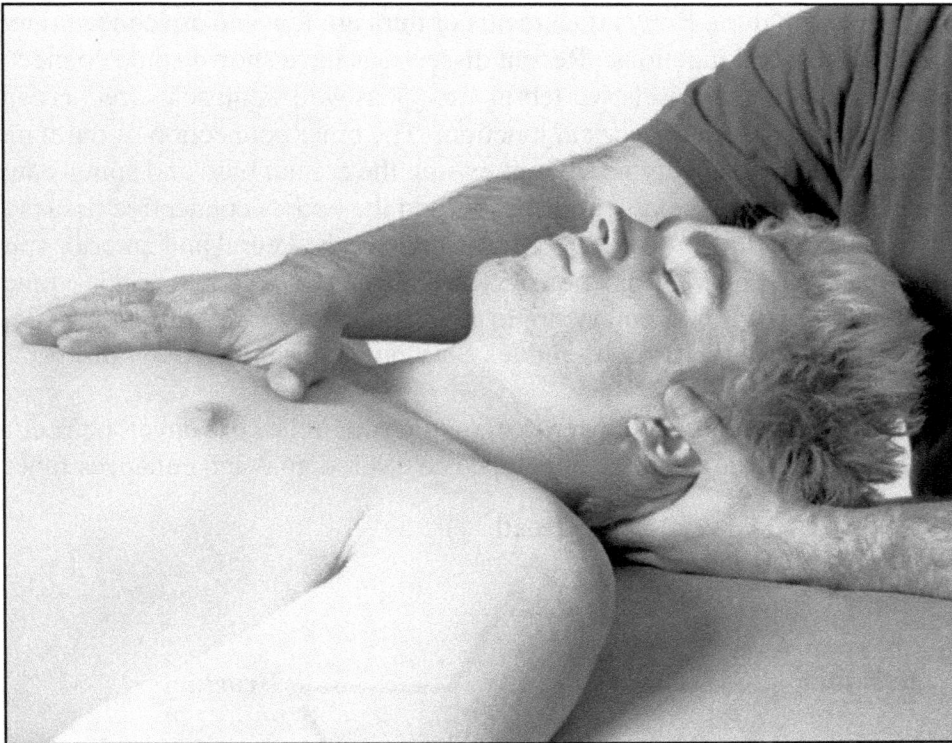

Occipitosternal Axis Treatment

CRANIOFASCIAL CONTINUITY AND THE CORE ENVELOPE

Fascia invests every tissue and every cavity in the body. Bone, cartilage, ligament, tendon, muscle, nerve, vessel, and organ all have fascial layers contributing to their structure and associated function. Cellular interstitial space, basement membranes, and lamina intima are all specializations of fascia with important physiologic relations. In the brain, the dural meninges function as the connective tissue investing the central nervous system.

Functional connections between cranial and fascial elements are many. Midline fluid dynamics, suspended automatically shifting fulcrums, and respiratory phase influences are a few examples. But where do the structural dural and fascial compartments of the body actually connect? Because of the bony calvarium and vertebral column there are few interconnections between the dural meninges and the rest of the body's connective tissues. Tendon and ligamentous structures interface with these bony structures but not with dura. Bony attachments of dura are few and are concentrated at the craniocervical and lumbosacral junctions. Recent dissections have shown some connections between dural meninges and blood vessels (vertebral artery), as well as muscles (rectus capitus posterior minor) concentrated at the craniocervical junction. The other connection of dural meninges is in the investing sheath surrounding every nerve root exiting the cranial base and spinal canal. The greatest interconnection between these neural sheaths and the body's connective tissues occurs at the sympathetic nerve ganglia and plexus of nerves formed along the lateral and anterior spinal column and at the brachial and sciatic nerve projections. Nerve plexuses also correspond to functional organizational relations derived from embryologic development. We call this craniofascial interface the core envelope. Its symmetrical form resembles a six-pointed star (see diagram).

The relationship between the upper and lower extremity through the core envelope is clinically important. Balanced tissue throughout the envelope is a desired goal and enhances functional responses throughout the body.

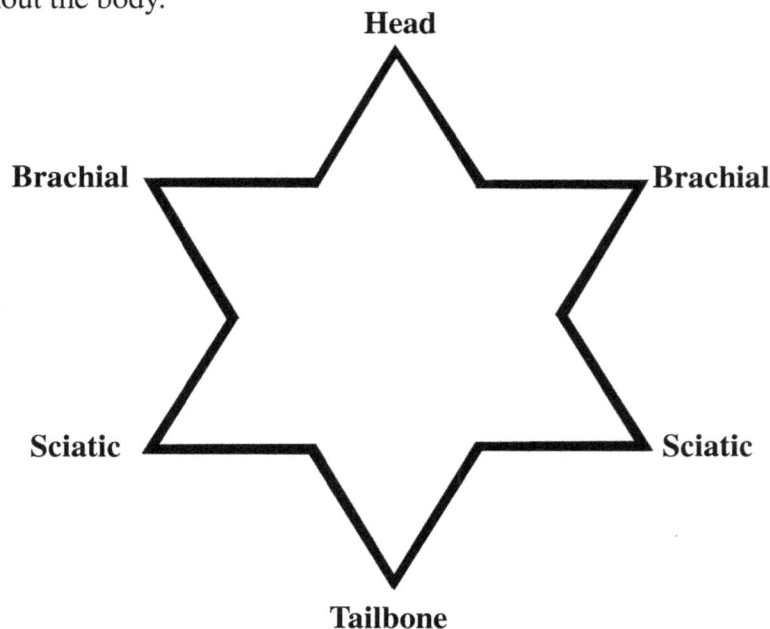

Geometric Structure of the Core Envelope

CORE ENVELOPE RELEASE

Based on osteopathic approaches developed by Jean- Pierre Barral D.O. (UK)

Dural-Vertebrobasilar Artery Interface

Diagnosis: With the operator sitting at the head of the patient the occiput is held bilaterally just posterior to the condyles. Traction is introduced one side at a time in a posterior-medial direction (sidebending away) with slight rotation in the opposite direction (towards). The relative compliance of suboccipital tissues to this traction is compared left to right. The side with more tension is restricted.

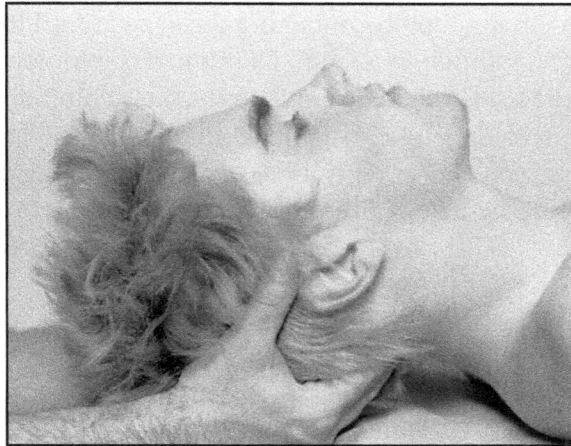

Dural-Vertebrobasilar Artery Interface Diagnosis

Treatment is by direct dural stretching with sidebending away and rotation towards the restricted side. Contact is made on the inferior occiput with one hand and the cervicothoracic junction/ first rib of the same side with the other hand. The cervicothoracic junction/ first rib is stabilized while cephalad traction is applied to the occiput during the flexion phase of the CRI. Traction is partially released during extension then re-applied during flexion until a stretching release is palpated between the two hands. Posterior-medial traction is then re-tested for symmetry.

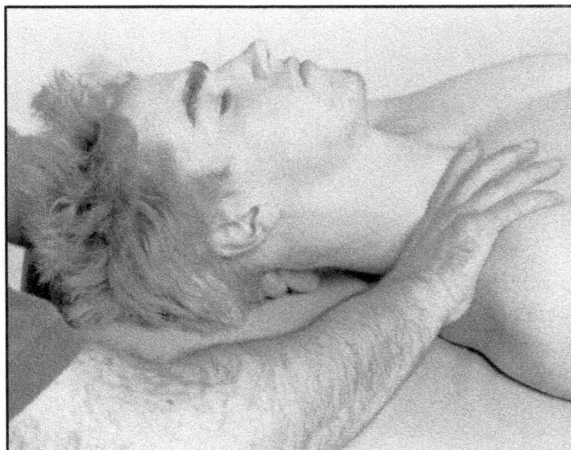

Dural-Vertebrobasilar Artery Interface Treatment

Brachial Sheath

Diagnosis: With the operator at the head of the supine patient, craniofascial tension of the brachial sheath can be palpated deep in the anterior cervical region, just posterior to the posterior head of the sternocleidomastoid tendon, between the anterior and medial scalenes. Nerve fibers within the sheath can be palpated as "strings" and an area of tension appreciated by compression along its width with the thumb. Comparison can be made from left to right to note relative amounts of sheath tension.

Treatment, Phase I: With the operator's palpating hand on the patient's shoulder, the thumb maintains sheath contact while the other hand slips under the patient's cervical spine contacting the ipsilateral lamina between the spinous and transverse processes. Several cervical segments are tested in response to slight traction with the thumb contacting the sheath until the segment demonstrating the most response (i.e tension) or stretch, is found. Continued rhythmic traction is introduced at this level by pushing the patient's shoulder caudad and then medial, maintaining thumb contact on the point of tension within the sheath. Traction is applied and then released repeatedly until sheath tension is resolved. Medial traction should be initiated only when caudad traction produces a slight relaxation response. Care should be taken in the cervical contact to not overstretch the nerve sheath during the medial traction phase. Slight reduction in cervical counterforce may be helpful.

Treatment, Phase II: While maintaining thumb contact on the brachial plexus, the operator shifts to sit beside the patient on the side of the dysfunction. The operator's free hand slides under the shoulder into the axilla to locate the exiting nerve sheaths, locating points of tension by applying traction through the arm and observing for motion under the thumb. Points of tension are treated by rhythmic application and release of arm traction until sheath tension is resolved. Resolution is perceived as a distal gliding of the nerve sheath at both the neck and arm contacts. Similar points of nerve sheath tension can be located and treated along the entire arm and forearm.

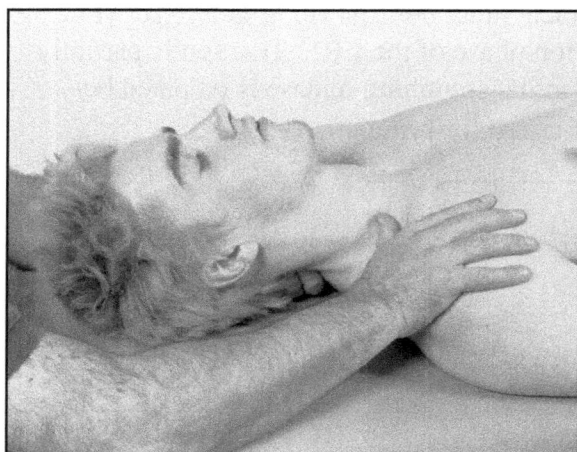

Brachial Sheath Treatment,
Phase I

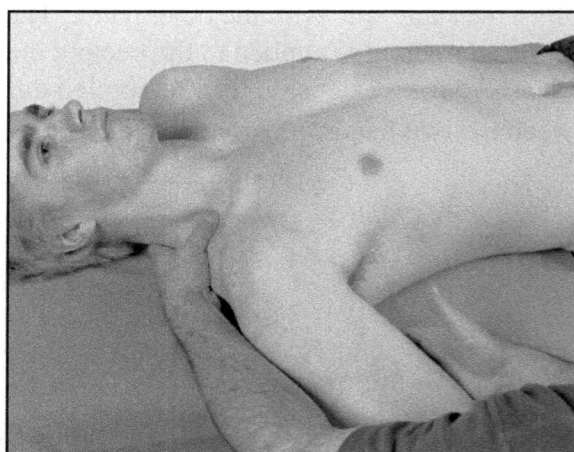

Brachial Sheath Treatment,
Phase II

Sciatic Sheath

Diagnosis: Tension of the sciatic sheath can be palpated high in the ischiorectal fossa below the piriformis muscle in the sciatic notch. The ipsilateral sciatic sheath should always be treated if the brachial sheath is restricted.

Treatment, Phase I: Standing at the patient's side, the operator's cephalad hand contacts the sciatic sheath with the 2nd and 3rd fingers, one on top of the other. The operator's caudad forearm supports the patient's leg introducing hip flexion, external rotation, abduction and returning to the midline with hip extension, adduction, and internal rotation. During the flexion/abduction movement, the nerve sheath is tractioned inferolaterally; during hip extension/adduction, the sheath is tractioned inferomedially. Release is felt as a caudad glide of the sciatic sheath.

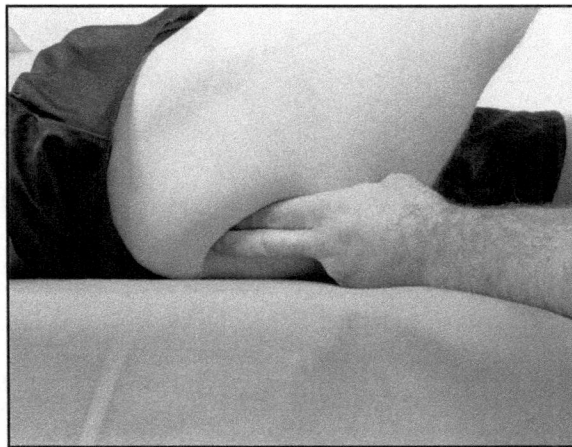

Sciatic Sheath Treatment Hand Contact

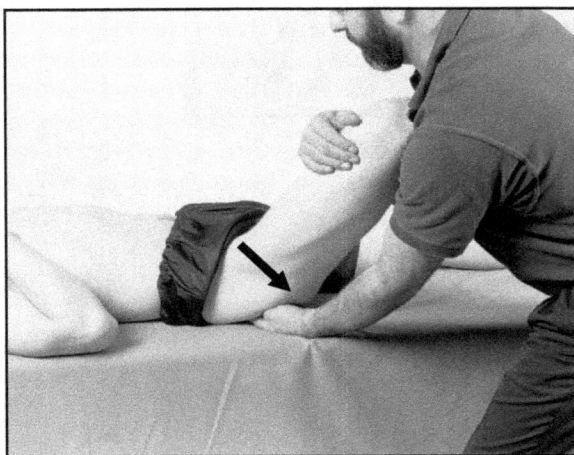

Sciatic Sheath Treatment , Phase I
Flexion/Abduction With Lateral Traction

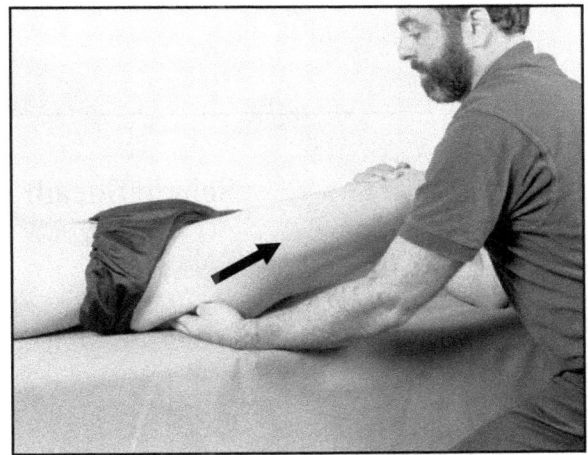

Sciatic Sheath Treatment , Phase I
Extension/Adduction With Medial Traction

Treatment, Phase II: Operator sits on the table facing the patient, with the patient's leg supported on the operator's shoulder. The operator's thumbs find the sciatic nerve sheath in the lower buttock between the hamstring fibers, locating areas of tension as thumbs track distally. Areas of tension are held beneath the thumbs as the operator leans back, extending the patient's knee, stretching the thigh and the associated sciatic nerve sheath. Nerve sheath tracking to locate areas of tension may proceed to the patient's ankle.

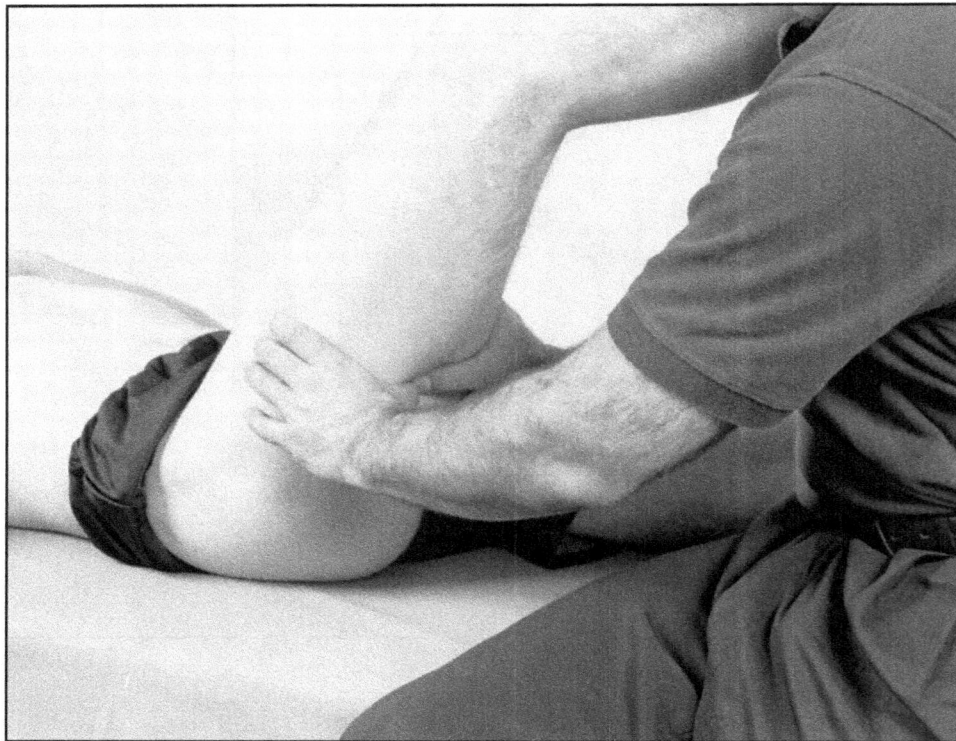

Sciatic Sheath Treatment , Phase II

UPPER EXTREMITY RELEASE

Based on osteopathic approaches developed by Dr. Anthony Chila, D.O., F.A.A.O.

A. General Considerations

1. Myofascial-ligamentous release of the upper extremity will apply the concepts of torsion, traction, leverage, and rhythm with respiratory cooperation. This release of the upper extremity is a comprehensive procedure incorporating a dynamic interplay between operator and patient. Deliberate movement is performed in rhythmic progression in conjunction with respiratory cooperation, facilitating fascial-ligamentous balance, neuromuscular release, and neuromuscular re-education. The result is greater freedom and efficiency of motion of the upper extremity in relation to both central neurologic and circulatory mechanisms.

2. The procedure encourages articulating full ranges of motion with alternating movements away from and toward the midline. The response in the tissues being palpated is noted as to the directions that create a sense of ease and the directions that increase tension. The process is guided toward increasing movement into the directions and positions of ease, synchronizing with respiration and controlling the rhythm of movement for optimal patient responses. Motion is constant, occasionally returning to positions of previous restriction to monitor efficacy of release.

3. Performed in a sidelying position, operator facing the patient, manipulative interventions of the upper extremity are directed in a dynamic process from one region to the next in a fluid pattern of motion and release. The following regions become the focus for successive upper extremity release:

   a. cervicothoracic spine

   b. medial scapulothoracic articulation

   c. anterior and posterior axilla

   d. thoracolumbar junction and lower costal cage

   e. clavicular and glenohumeral articulations

   f. wrist, hand, and fingers

   g. superior thoracic aperture.

B. Procedure for Upper Extremity Release

1. <u>Cervicothoracic Spine</u>

The entire sequence for myofascial-ligamentous release of the upper extremity begins in the central axis of the body. Varying degrees of leverage are exerted through the cervical and cervicothoracic regions. This is accomplished by the operator's passive induction of flexion, extension, bilateral side-bending and rotation through the patient's head. The impact of the variable leverages is monitored at successively lower levels of the cervicothoracic column and paravertebral regions. This initial preparation helps to reduce tension throughout the cervical and thoracic regions which may contribute to restriction of motion of the upper extremity.

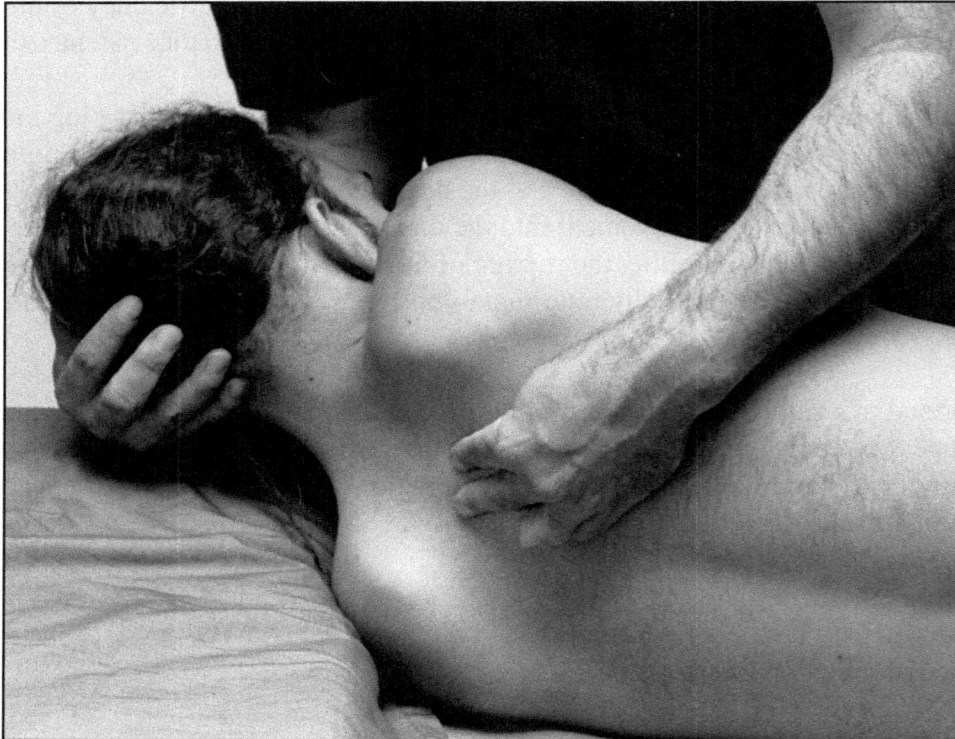

Cervicothoracic Spine Treatment

2. Medial Scapulothoracic Articulation

The scapula is identified and isolated by full use of the fingers and thumbs of both hands of the operator. The extended fingers spread throughout the medial border from the superior to the inferior spines, and the thumbs contact the lateral border of the scapula. The abducted shoulder is placed over the operator's cephalad forearm. Release of scapulofascial restriction is accomplished by the operator's passive induction of motion laterally, medially, cephalad, caudad, clockwise and counterclockwise. The direction and amount of resistance is determined by testing each plane of motion. Direct release or indirect, respiratory-assisted release of restricted motion helps to mobilize the scapula on the posterior thorax.

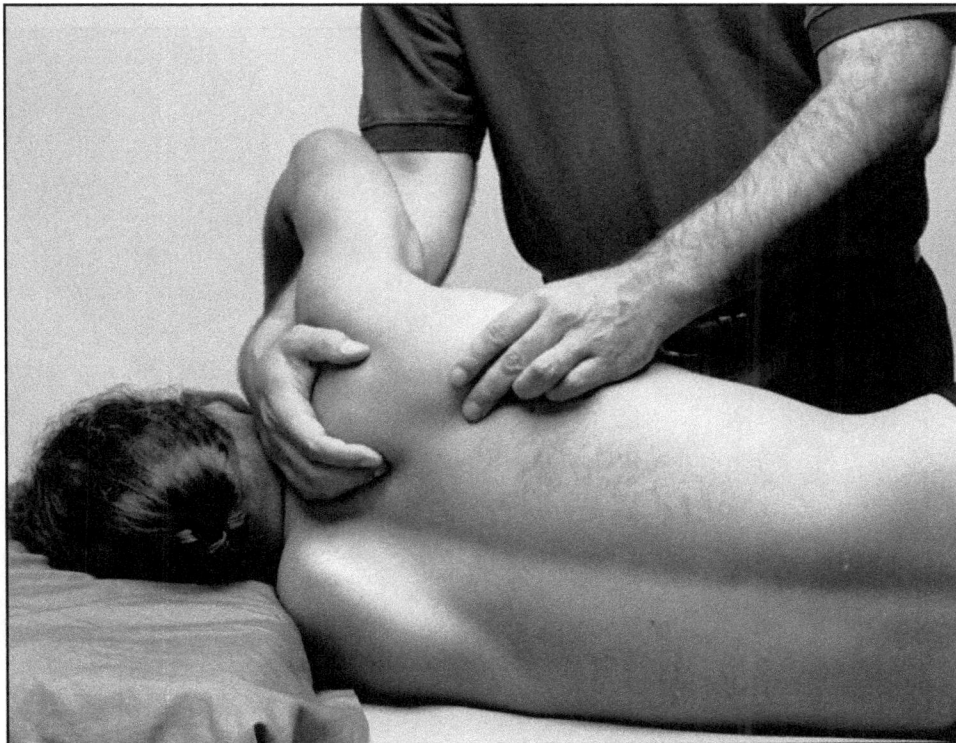

Medial Scapulothoracic Articulation Treatment

3. **Anterior and Posterior Axilla (Gateway to the Upper Extremity)**

The operator strips the muscular and fascial tissues of the anterior axilla, passively lifting the muscular and fascial tissues of the pectoral area anteriorly and cephalad while simultaneous motion is introduced into the patient's pronated arm in a posterolateral direction.

For the posterior axilla the muscular and fascial tissues are passively stripped in a cephalad direction while simultaneously directing the upper extremity with the other hand in a superior medial direction with forearm supination. The operator switches hand contact as he moves between the two release positions. In both instances, the patient's arm is lifted vertically in order to facilitate axillary decongestion. The patient's wrist is pronated to facilitate release of the pectoral area and supinated to facilitate release of the posterior axillary area.

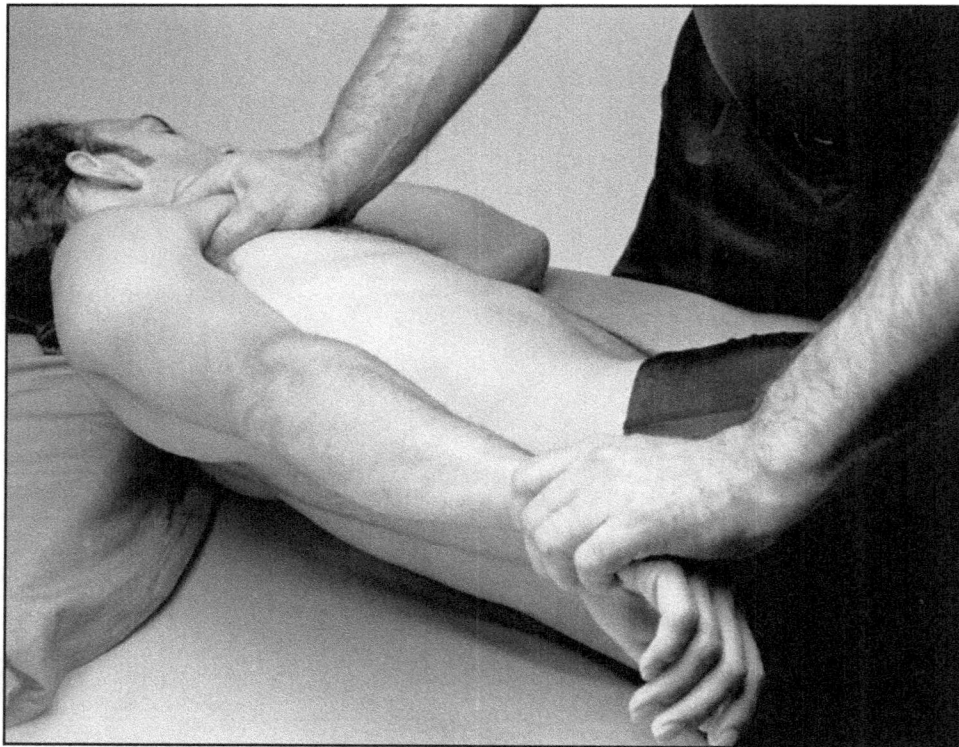

Anterior Axilla Treatment

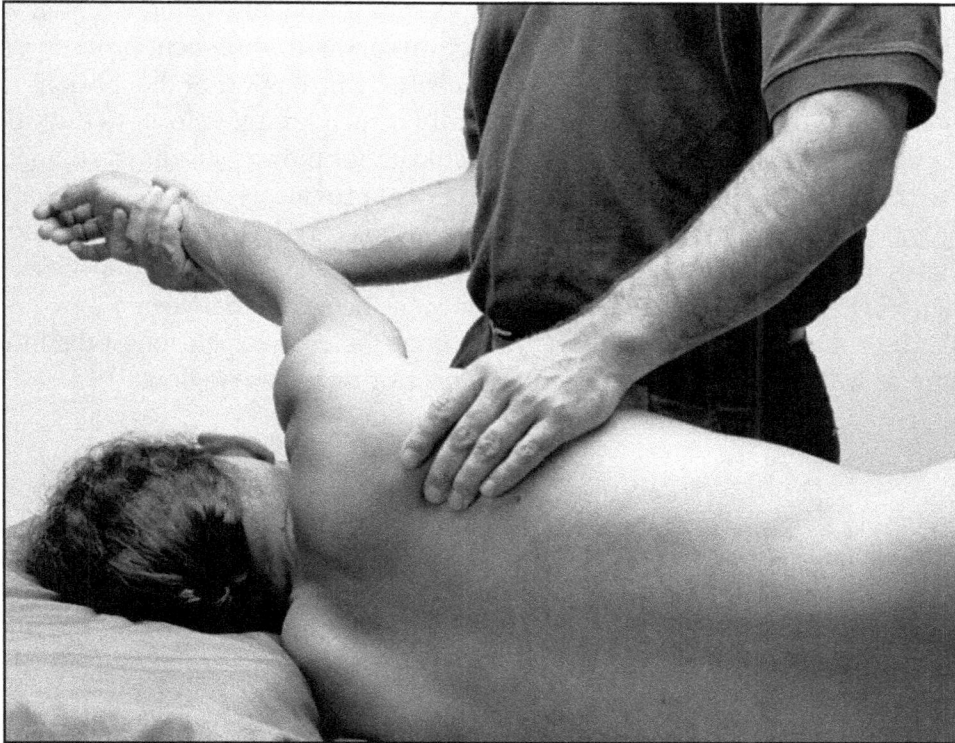

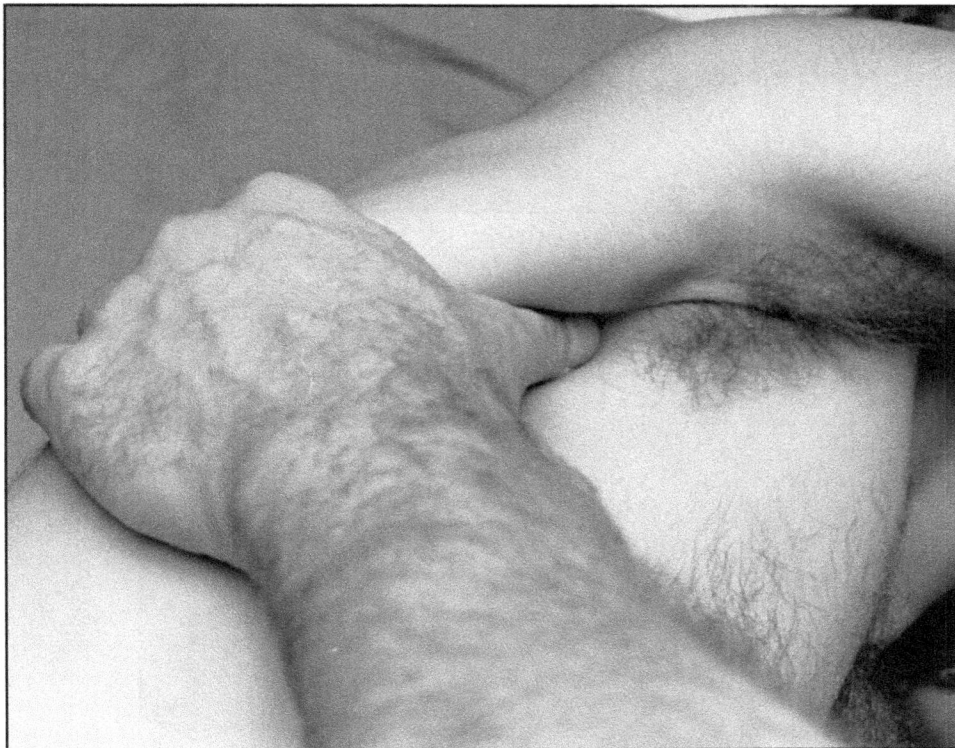

Posterior Axilla Treatment

4. Thoracolumbar Junction and Lower Costal Cage

This is accomplished by the physician's support of the patient's elbow region with one hand and the wrist region with the other hand. For this and all subsequent procedures, the fulcrum is established by the elbows of the physician's body in support of the motions of the patient's upper extremity. The extended upper extremity is then brought closer to the side of the body. As the upper extremity is carried toward the posterior thorax, sustained supination facilitates release of the thoracolumbar junction. The patient provides assistance by inhalation. Alternately, sustained pronation as the upper extremity is carried toward the xiphoid process facilitates myofascial release along the lower costal cage. The patient provides assistance by exhalation. The operator switches hand contact as he moves between the two release positions. The cumulative effect of these forces contributes to expansion of the inferior thoracic aperture as well as ligamentous articular release of the elbow region.

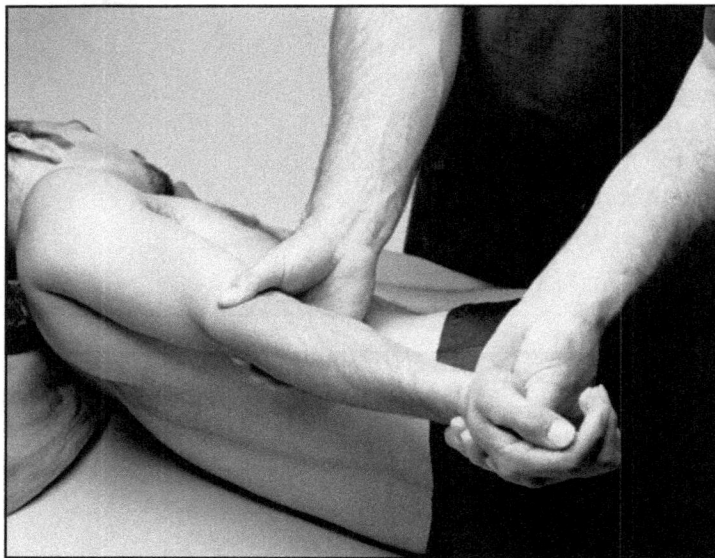

Thoracolumbar Junction Treatment (Supination)

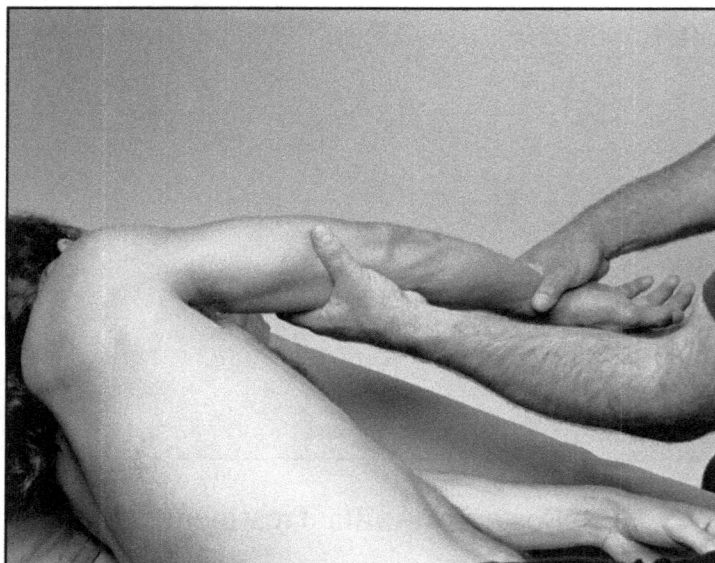

Lower Costal Cage Treatment (Pronation)

5. Clavicular and Glenohumeral Articulations

Release for this region is accomplished by repeating the motions previously described with more abduction so that forces are transmitted into the distal clavicle and glenohumeral region. Continue with sustained supination as the upper extremity is carried toward the posterior thorax facilitating release of the acromioclavicular articulation and the glenohumeral regions. The patient provides assistance by inhalation. Sustained pronation as the upper extremity is carried toward the manubrial region facilitates release of the manubrial area and the sterno-clavicular articulation. The patient provides assistance by exhalation. Additional traction can be applied by flexing the elbow and using this leverage to increase distractive forces into the glenohumeral and clavicular areas.

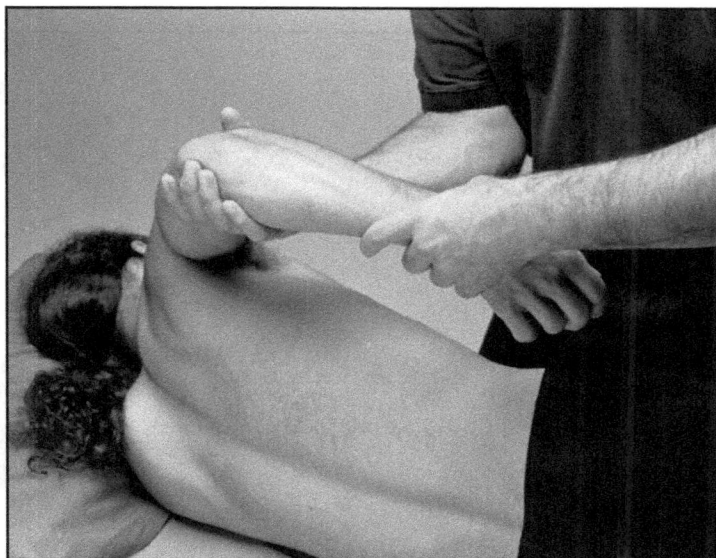

Glenohumeral Treatment (Supination)

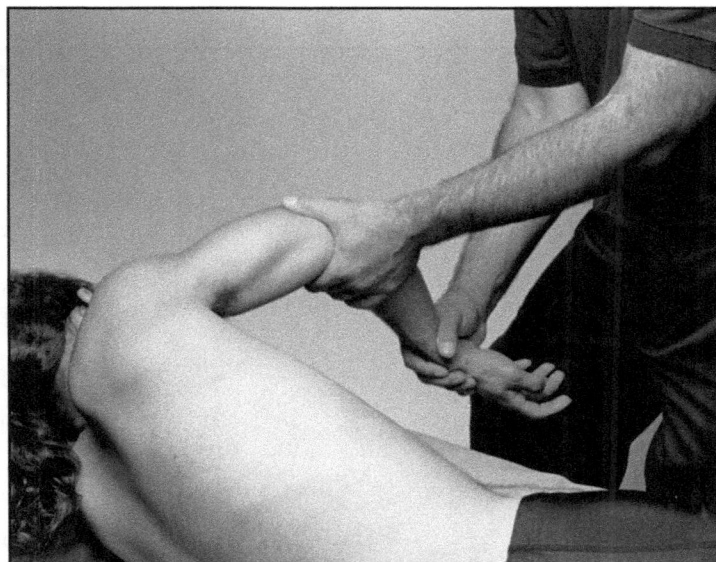

Clavicular Treatment (Pronation)

6. **Wrist, Hand and Finger Articulations**

This is accomplished by sustained, alternating supination and pronation which facilitates the release of myofascial-ligamentous tension along the course of the interosseous membrane to the flexor retinaculum. The addition of alternating flexion and extension of the wrist facilitates the release of articular dysfunctions of the carpal bones. Myofascial and fascial-ligamentous release of the palmar area precedes articulatory release of the small joints of the fingers and thumb. The progress of the sequence is from the small finger to the thumb. Operator palpatory perception of releasing responses should be noted either in conjunction with movement away from the midline or toward the midline. Once noted, directions of ease should be preferentially directed into the releasing position for each area of dysfunction.

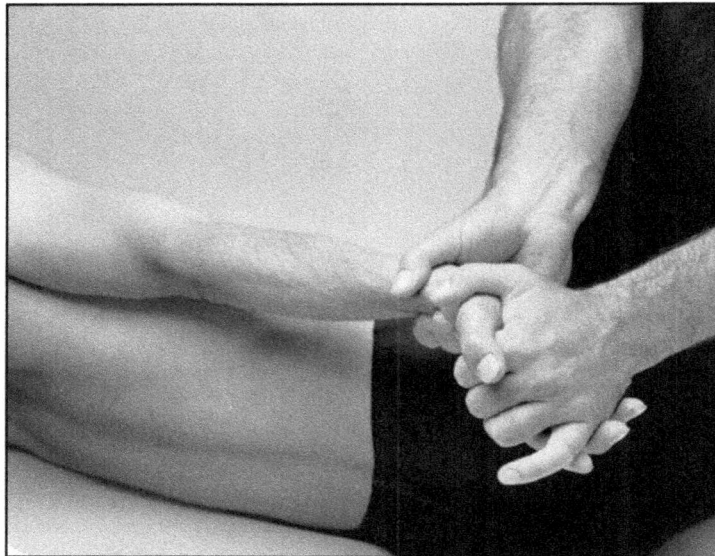

Wrist Articulation Treatment Supination Phase

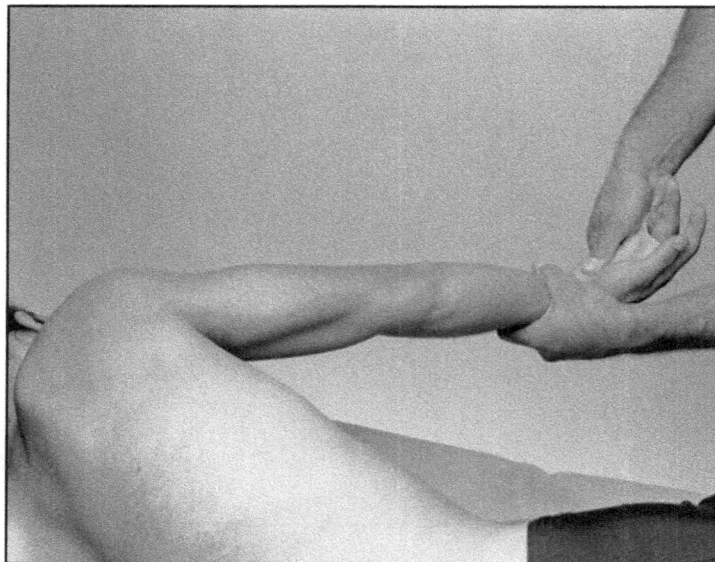

Wrist Articulation Treatment Pronation Phase

7. <u>Superior Thoracic Aperture (Exit From the Upper Extremity)</u>

This is accomplished by grasping the deep webbing between the index finger and thumb of the patient's extended upper extremity. In acupuncture, this is known as the Hoku point (Colon 4). Sustained, alternating supination and pronation facilitates the release of congestion in this area and contributes to release of the cervicothoracic junction.

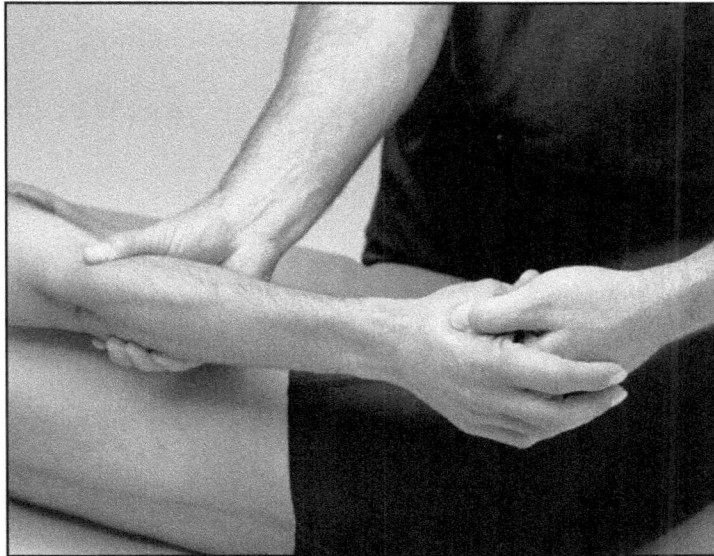

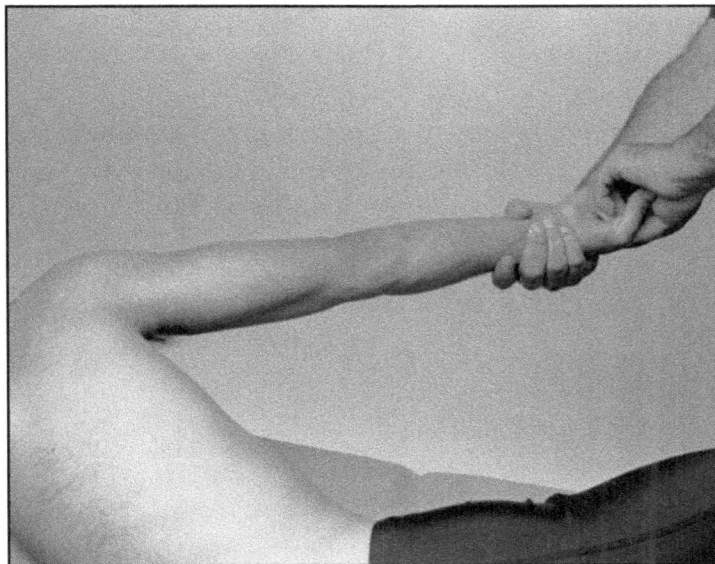

Superior Thoracic Aperture Treatment

LOWER EXTREMITY RELEASE
Based on osteopathic approaches developed
by Anthony Chila, D.O., F.A.A.O.

A. General Considerations

1. The application of myofascial-ligamentous release principles will be applied to the concepts of torsion, traction, leverage, and rhythm in the lower extremities.

2. Manipulative intervention by a physician performing this procedure is directed to the following areas of the body:

   a. Lower Leg:

      i. <u>Valgus (Abduction) Phase</u>. Lower leg positions are introduced in a therapeutic process where areas of ligamentous release (ease) and tension are established in the following paired structures (area of ease/area of tension):

         (a) medial/lateral malleolus

         (b) lateral/medial knee

         (c) medial thigh/tensor fasciae latae

         (d) inguinal area/trochanter

      ii. <u>Varus (Adduction) Phase</u>. Lower leg positions are introduced in a therapeutic process where areas of ligamentous release (ease) and tension are established in the following paired structures (area of ease/area of tension):

         (a) lateral/medial malleolus

         (b) medial/lateral knee

         (c) tensor fasciae latae/medial thigh

         (d) trochanter/inguinal area

B. Procedure for Lower Extremity Release

1. General Considerations

Procedures are performed with the patient supine, selecting the lower extremity demonstrating greatest tension in response to myofascial screening tests of the lower extremities. Torsion, traction and leverage are selectively employed in two phases to release muscular, connective tissue and articular dysfunction. The fulcrum is established by the physician's use of the elbows of both arms in supporting the motions of the patient's foot, lower leg, and knee.

2. **Lower Leg: Valgus (Abduction) Phase**

The plantar surface of the foot is inverted and plantar flexed. Torsion is introduced between the lateral ankle and the knee. The effect of torsion is steadily advanced by slowly moving the knee medially, resulting in progressive abduction of the lower leg. Torsion will be felt in the lateral malleolar area, the medial compartmental area of the knee, the tensor fasciae latae area, and the trochanter. Conversely, fascial ligamentous release or relaxation will be appreciated in the medial thigh, medial malleolus, lateral knee and inguinal areas. Additional release of the ankle and knee can be appreciated with gradual movement of the knee away from the midline and the hip into extension, bringing the foot and lower leg below the plane of the table. Gradual increase in knee flexion can be better accomplished in this position with additional release of the lower leg and ankle. Upon completion of this phase, the lower extremity is gradually extended and slowly returned to the tabletop.

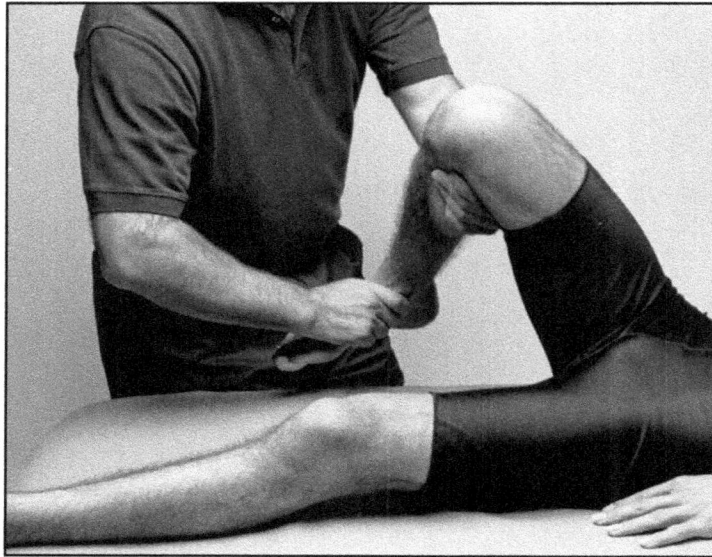

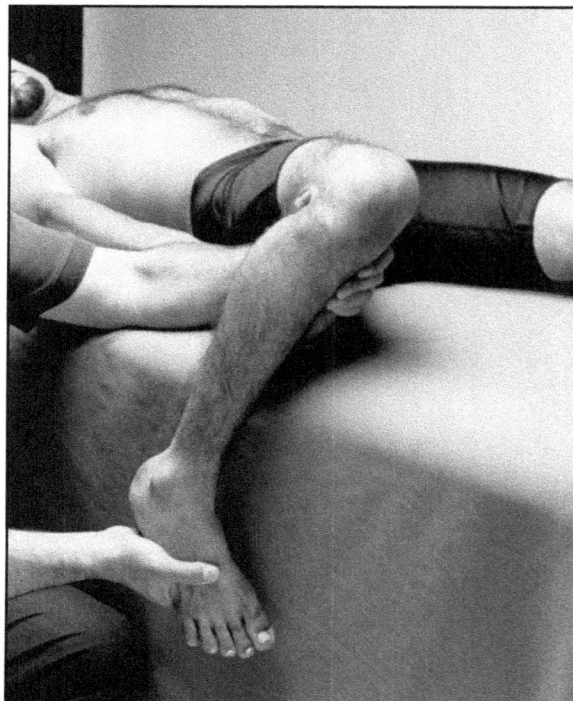

Valgus (Abduction) Phase of Lower Leg Treatment

Release of the hindfoot and forefoot, as well as tarsal elements, can be accomplished by the operator supporting the popliteal area on his flexed upper arm/elbow while grasping with two hands the restricted elements in the ankle/foot. Restricted elements can be positioned in the direction of ease in order to facilitate their release in this position.

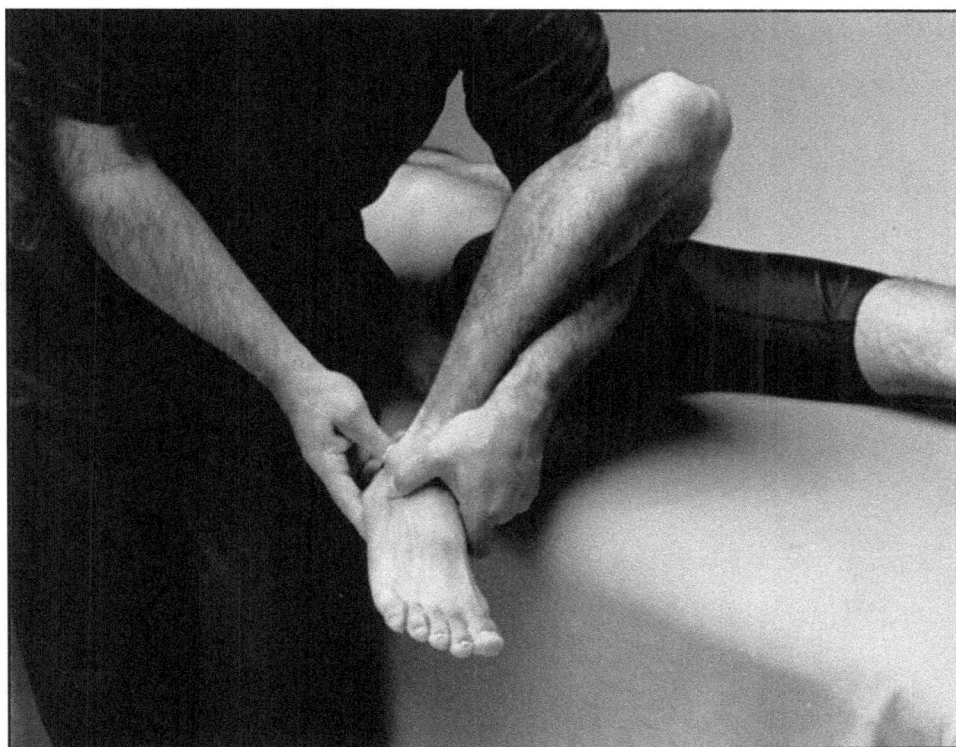

Ankle/Foot Treatment- Valgus Phase

3. Lower Leg: Varus (Adduction) Phase

The plantar surface of the foot is everted and dorsiflexed. Torsion is introduced between the medial ankle and the knee. The effect of torsion is steadily advanced by slowly moving the knee away from the midline, resulting in progressive adduction of the lower leg and abduction and external rotation of the hips. The heel is progressively brought closer to the pube. The torsion will be felt in the medial malleolar area, the lateral compartmental area of the knee, the medial thigh, and inguinal areas. Fascial ligamentous relaxation will be appreciated in the lateral malleolar area, the medial compartment of the knee, the tensor fascia latae and trochanter area. Upon completion of this phase, the lower extremity is gradually extended and slowly returned to the tabletop.

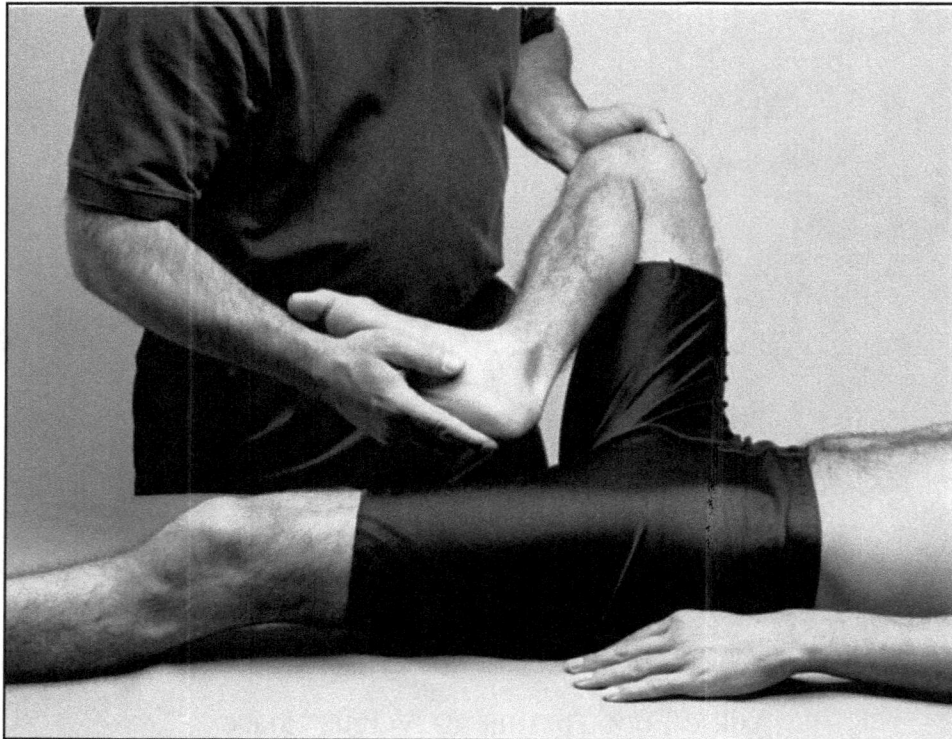

Varus (Adduction) Phase of Lower Leg Treatment

Positioning of the operator's flexed elbow in the popliteal area can allow for bilateral hand contact of the <u>ankle and foot</u>. Restricted areas responding with increasing ease to this positioning can be monitored for maximum relaxation and release.

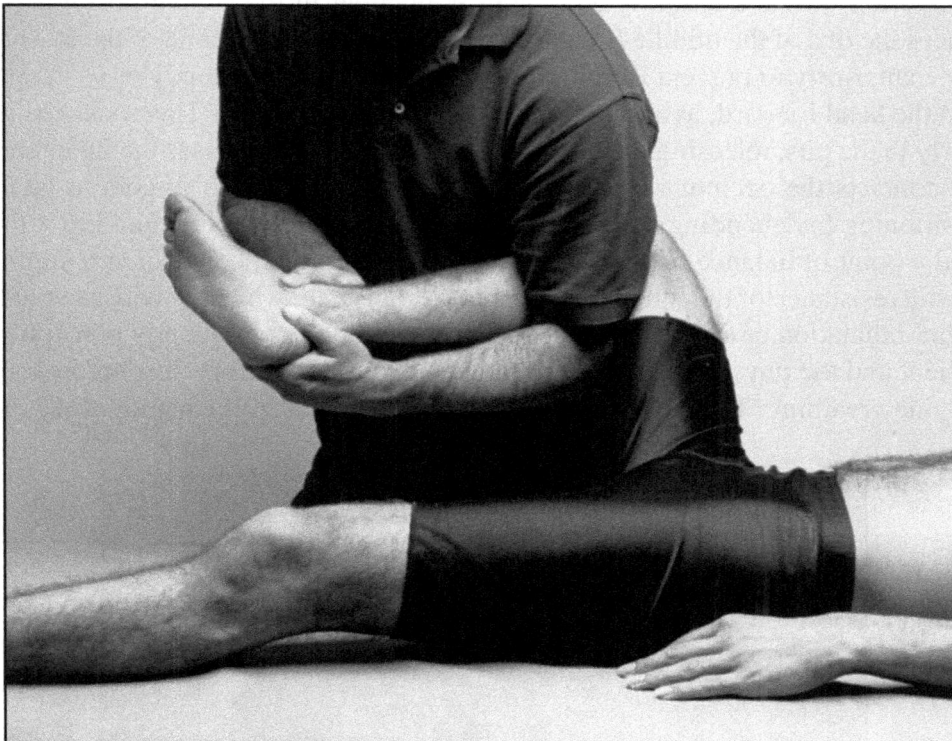

Ankle/Foot Treatment-Varus Phase

OSTEOPATHIC TECHNIQUE OF WILLIAM G. SUTHERLAND, D.O.

A. Osseous Techniques.

1. Condyloatlantal Articulation

   a. The articular pits of the atlas converge anteriorly and inferiorly and they curve cranialward to a position anterior to the occipital condyles. The motion permitted is a nodding of the head as the condyles rock forward and back in the cup-shaped pits of the atlas.

   b. Correction of dysfunction is done with the patient in the supine position. The physician places the tips of the middle fingers against the posterior tubercle of the atlas and holds that bone anteriorly to prevent it from moving dorsally with the condyles as the patient nods or tips the head forward, avoiding flexion of the cervical spine. This rocks the occiput posteriorly in the pits, releasing the condyles from the atlas, and tenses the ligaments. The operator contacts the occiput with the tips of the third and fourth fingers to facilitate optimal positioning (sidebending and rotation) of the occiput. The right and left articulations will find a point of balance between them, perceptible to the physician as a slight springing or elastic resistance of the ligaments. This position is held while the patient holds the breath in either inhalation or exhalation. Release of the fixation is frequently perceptible to both the patient and the physician, usually during the respiratory efforts just before the patient must resume breathing. This approach is effective regardless of the nature of the dysfunction.

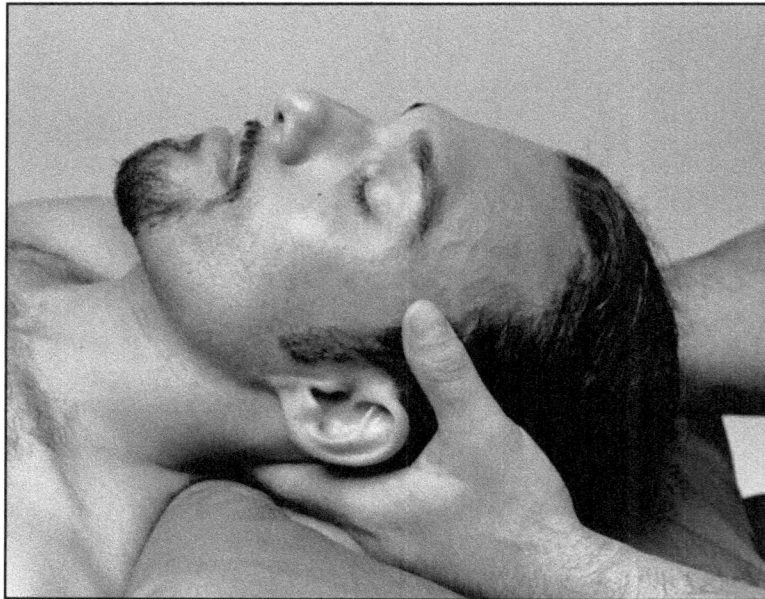

Treatment of Condyloatlantal Articulation

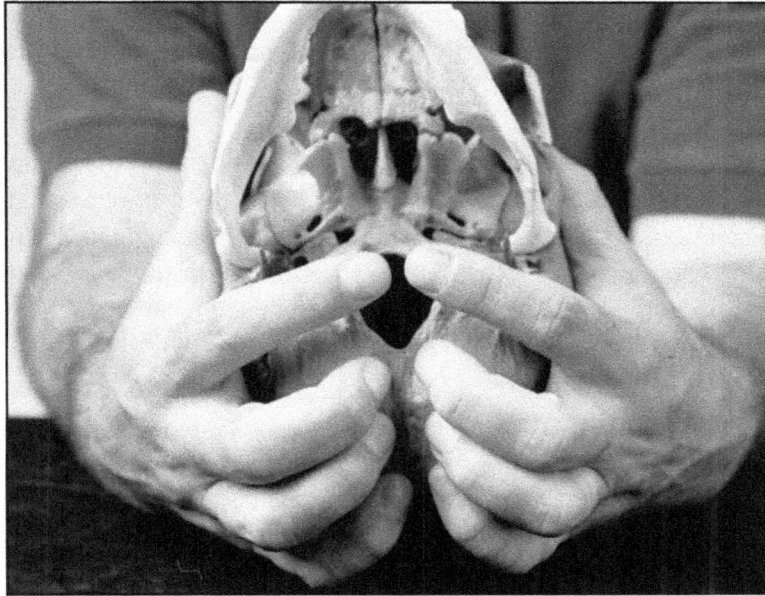

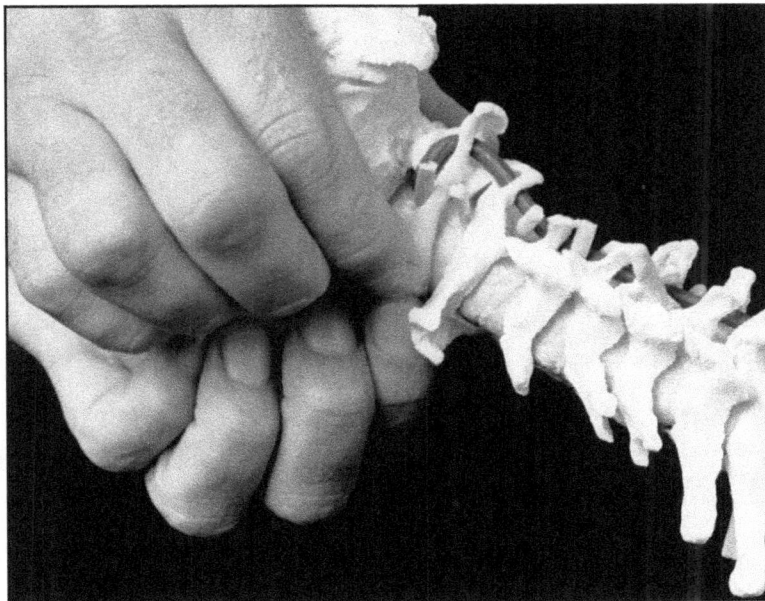

Anatomical Hand Positioning for Treatment of Condyloatlantal Articulation

2. Rib Articulation

a. Dysfunction of ribs is considered as an articular strain of the capsular, radiate and interarticular ligaments connecting the head of the rib to the bodies of the vertebrae. Diagnosis of a rib dysfunction can be made by gently palpating over the lateral aspect of the ribs until a rib demonstrating reduced compliance is palpated. This rib is contacted along its lateral aspect with the thumbs and the anterior and posterior aspects with the fingertips. Motion testing is carried out to determine if the rib moves more easily in anterior or posterior direction.

   1. For a rib that is moving more easily in a <u>posterior</u> position, the operator will maintain the rib head in a posterior position as the patient is instructed to rotate slowly in the opposite direction. The patient is asked to inhale and exhale and hold the respiratory effort that produces greater relaxation of the rib. Additional fine-tuning movements of flexion or extension and side-bending can be used to maximize the fascial-ligamentous relaxation and release.

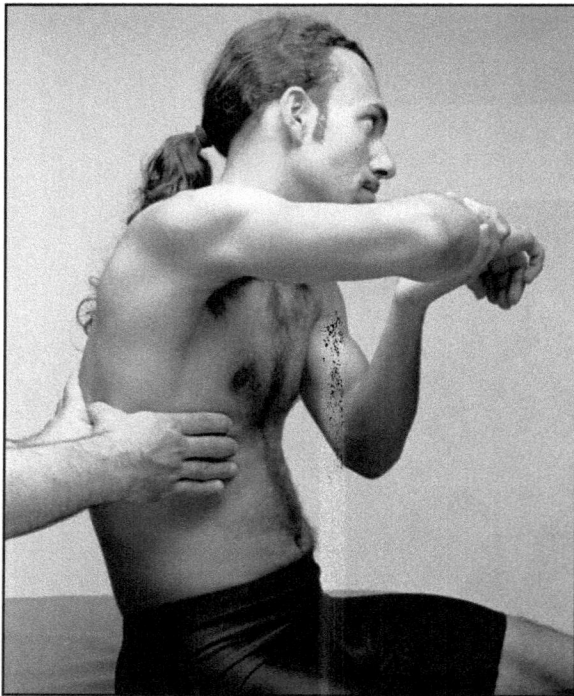

Hand Placement for
Posterior Rib Treatment

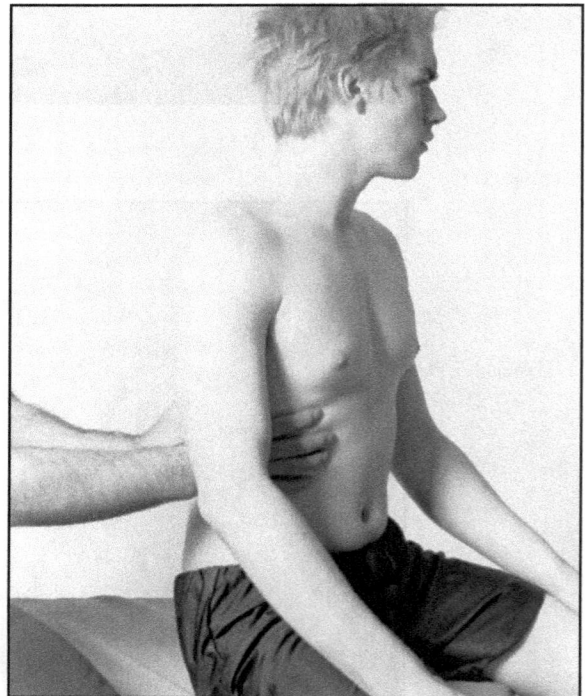

Treatment of a Posterior Rib

2. For a rib moving more easily in an <u>anterior</u> direction, the operator will stabilize the rib in an anterior relationship as the patient is instructed to rotate to the same side while assuming inhalation or exhalation assistance in the direction that produces greater relaxation. Additionally, fine-tuning of flexion, extension, and side-bending can also facilitate fascial-ligamentous relaxation and release.

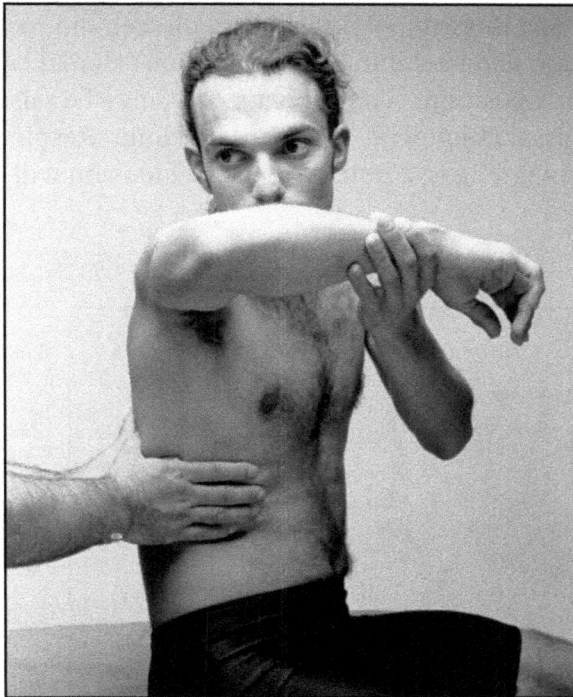

Hand Placement for
Anterior Rib Treatment

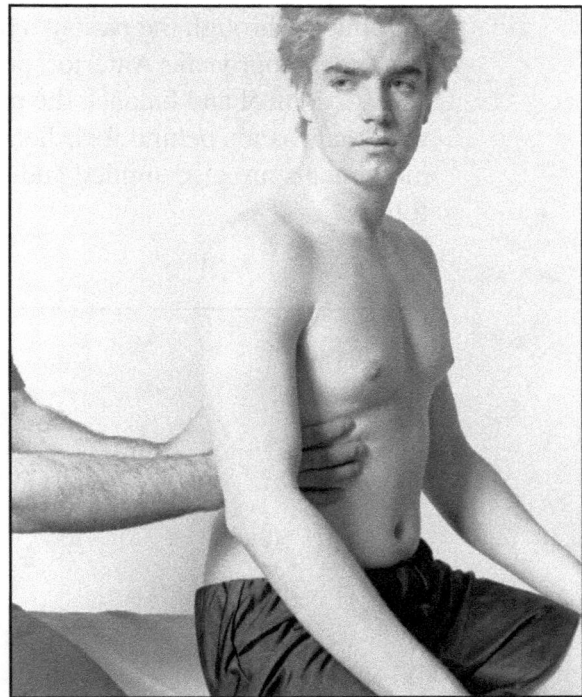

Treatment of an Anterior Rib

3. **Intraosseous Sternal Dysfunction**

a. Intrathoracic fascia and ligaments have relations transversely between anterior and posterior thoracic cage components. Internal structues associated with these fascia include heart, lung. esophagus, trachea, and major vessels. The sternum is the common attachment for these fascia anteriorly. Stress patterns are commonly introduced here due to ergonomic stresses and imbalances in respiratory (breathing) function. Adhesions from previous infectious processes in and around the lung may also influence fascial tensions and associated mobile functions. Rib dysfunctions should be addressed first to gain better access to these deeper intrathoracic structures.

b. Patient seated, operator standing behind the patient contacting an area of intraosseous sternal tension. Beginning with compression between the sternum and a counterpoint of posterior thoracic contact, passive and then active movements are introduced through the patient's head and thorax applying either a direcet, indirect or combined approach. Anterior, posterior, and lateral translatory motions should be used to control and balance the patient's position. The patient's arms may be raised with their hands behind their head in association with backward bending. Respiratory movements are also applied and an unwinding to a point of balanced tension will follow.

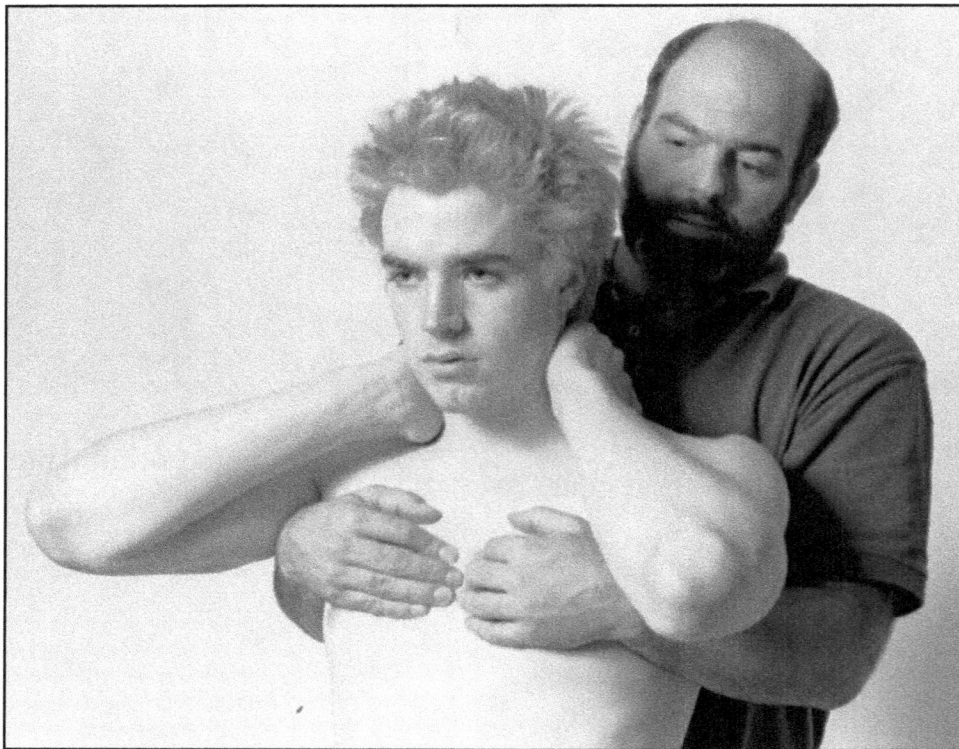

Treatment of Intraosseous Sternal Dysfunction

B. Non-Osseous Techniques

1. Anterior Cervical Fascia

a. The anterior cervical fascia is attached to the base of the skull, the mandible, hyoid, scapula, clavicle and sternum. Through the pretracheal fascia, it is connected with the fibrous pericardium, and thence with the diaphragm. It surrounds the pharynx, larynx and thyroid gland, it forms the carotid sheath, and by way of the prevertebral fascia is connected with that which surrounds the trachea and esophagus. The anterior cervical fascia, therefore, is concerned quite directly with lymphatic drainage of the head, neck, thorax and upper extremities. Not only voluntary movements, but respiratory activity is a factor in this vital function of the fascia, moving it forward in exhalation and backward in approximation to the spine during inhalation.

b. The "drag" on the cervical fascia is eliminated by having the patient seated, facing the physician. The patient's body is flexed and the head hangs forward. The physician directs the thumbs posteriorly and downward over the clavicles just lateral to the attachment of the sternomastoid muscles. With the arms placed lateral to those of the physician, the patient rests the hands on the physician's shoulders and slowly drops forward. This permits the physician's thumbs to advance into the mediastinal region, just anterior and to either side of the trachea. The operator will notice asymmetry in the tension of these fascial tissues, and direct the patient to side-bend and rotate in order to balance (relax) the tension palpated. The patient can be instructed to assume the respiratory phase that further relaxes these tissues. The physician approximates the thumbs enough to gently hold the pretracheal fascia while the patient slowly assumes the erect posture, but with the neck remaining in flexion (keep chin tucked). The patient is simultaneously instructed to release the breath being held. It is unnecessary to go so deep into the mediastinum as to cause discomfort to the patient. This technique lifts the fascia and reduces the "drag" from the contents of the costal cage.

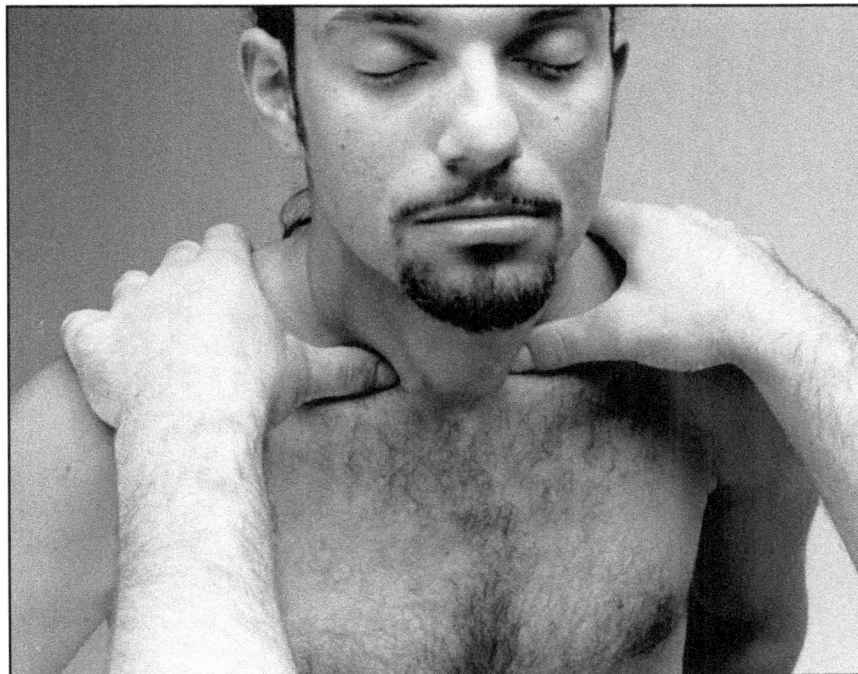

Hand Placement for Anterior Cervical Fascia Treatment

97

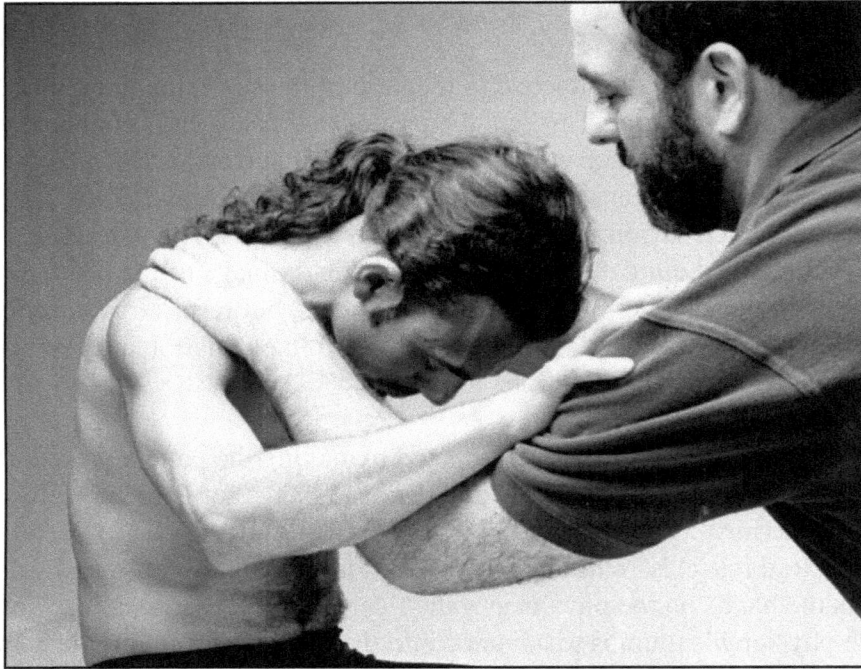

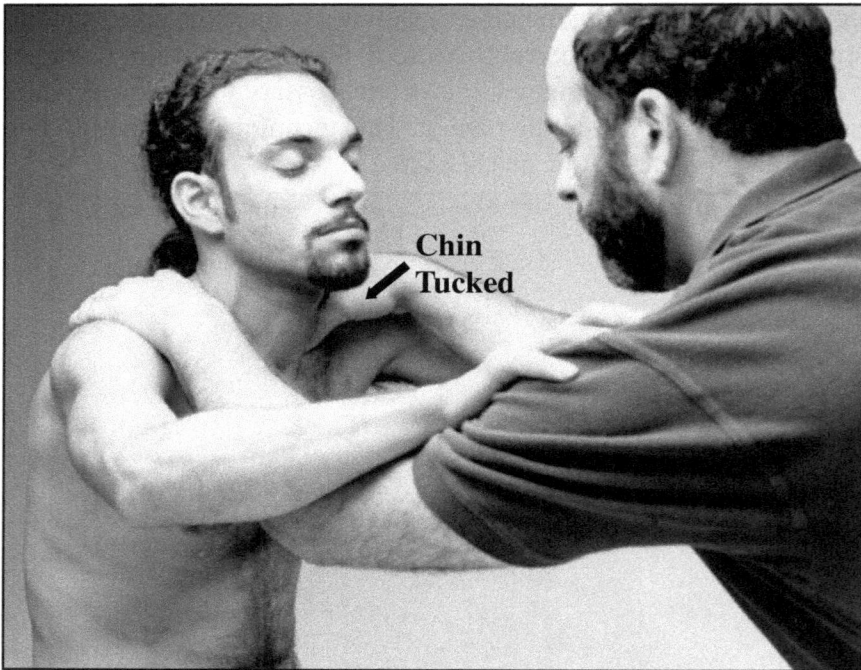

Chin
Tucked

Anterior Cervical Fascia Treatment

2. Diaphragm

a. Because of its relationships, the diaphragm deserves consideration other than as a muscle of respiration. The pericardium is firmly attached to it above, the peritoneum below, and the great vessels and esophagus pass through it. Being rather closely associated with the organs of respiration, circulation and digestion, it is important that the full excursion of the diaphragm be unimpeded. This is prevented by a "drag" on the abdominal fascia and may be restored by a technique known as the diaphragmatic lift. The object of the treatment is to draw the diaphragm cranially, elevating the floor of the thorax, drawing upward on the abdominal contents and promoting venous and lymphatic drainage from the lower half of the body. Visceroptosis and even internal hemorrhoids respond to this technique.

b. With patient supine, the physician introduces the fingertips under the costochondral, junctions. If the tone of the anterior diaphragm attachments are very high, then a specific release to address and relax this must be applied first (see Craniosacral, Part II). If contact in this area is particularly sensitive, the patient places their fingers under these junctions and the physician lifts on the patient's hands. As the patient exhales, the physician lifts the lower rim of the thorax in a cranial and slightly lateral direction. The advancement that is made is held during inspiration and is increased on exhalation. The patient is instructed not to hold the breath in, but to exhale immediately after inhalation. After several respiratory cycles, there is no further upward progress and the patient is told to breathe out, close the throat and attempt to expand the chest while pulling in the abdomen (sucking the abdominal contents towards the chest). This maneuver should be reviewed and practiced with the patient before starting the procedure to ensure proper execution.

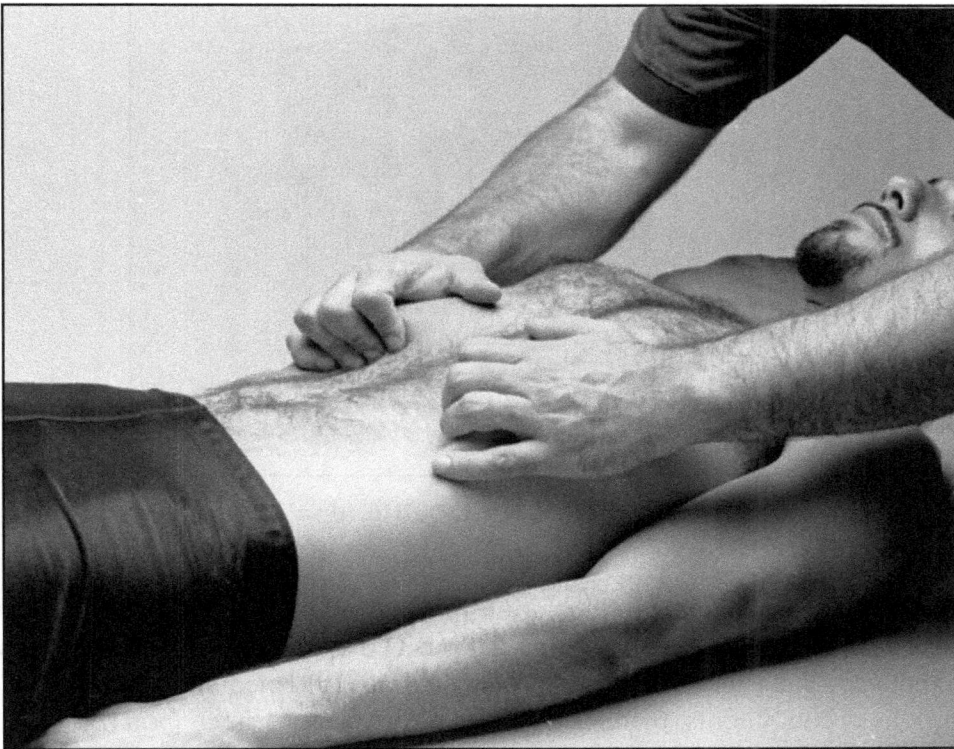

Diaphragm Treatment

3. Pelvic Lift

a. The fascial connections from the neck to the diaphragm have been mentioned. The direct attachment of the diaphragm to the liver, and the connections to the stomach, duodenum, psoas and peritoneum complete a chain embracing the viscera all the way down into the pelvis. Fascial "drag" has an adverse influence on the support and function of the organs and on the circulation and drainage of the lower half of the body. The aorta lies against the bodies of the vertebrae and is crossed anteriorly by the crura of the diaphragm. Thus the "drag" on the crura has a constricting effect upon the aorta, throwing an extra load upon the heart and predisposing to cardiac insufficiency.

b. An effective technique for reducing the "drag" on the fascia is applied with the patient lying on the left side. The thighs are straight or slightly flexed to the position in which the floor of the pelvis is most relaxed. The physician stands in back of the patient and starts the tips of the fingers medial to the right ischial tuberosity, advancing them upward between the obturator membrane and the rectum while the patient exhales. During inhalation the position of the fingers is held gently, but firmly, not allowing them to recede. This hand may be supported by the other hand to allow the fingers to hold more steadily and to note more carefully the resistance of the tissues. After several cycles of deep respiration, the resistance will be felt to diminish suddenly and the tissues spring upward in advance of the fingers.

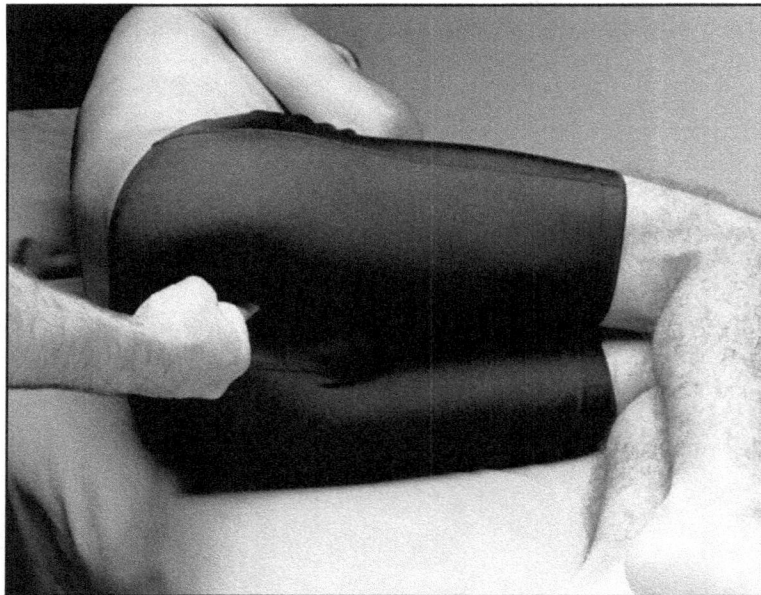

Pelvic Lift Treatment

c. This technique is adaptable to the various pelvic prolapses that are bound to cause a drag on the fascia and that persist partially because the support of that agency has been reduced. The fingers may be directed cranially and medially or anteriorly toward the cecum, uterus, bladder or prostate for specific effect upon those organs. It will be found easier and less uncomfortable to the patient than local treatment. If indicated, the technique may be applied to the left side of the pelvis.

4. **Popliteal Drainage**

  a. Movement of fluids from the popliteal space and below may be accelerated by drawing apart the tendons of the biceps and semi-tendinosus muscles, just above the knee. The patient is supine, with the knee flexed on the table or on the operator's shoulder (for additional hamstring stretch). The physician encircles the knee with both hands, using the fingertips for separation of the tendons. The patient alternately pulls their heel cephalad down into the table or operator's shoulder and then relaxes. The effort to flex the knee tends to compress the tissues of the popliteal space, which expands when the patient relaxes the leg and the physician separates the tendons. The effect is that of a booster pump in the return of the fluids toward the heart.

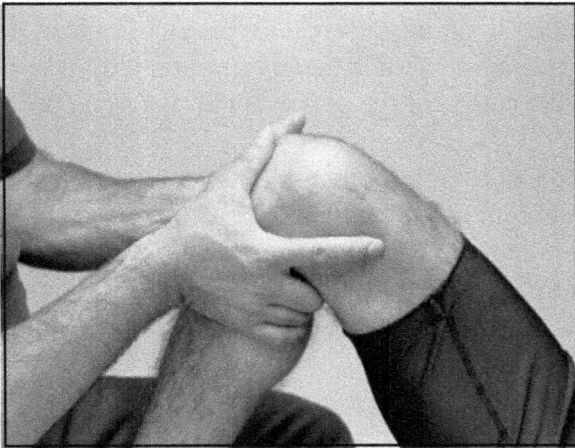

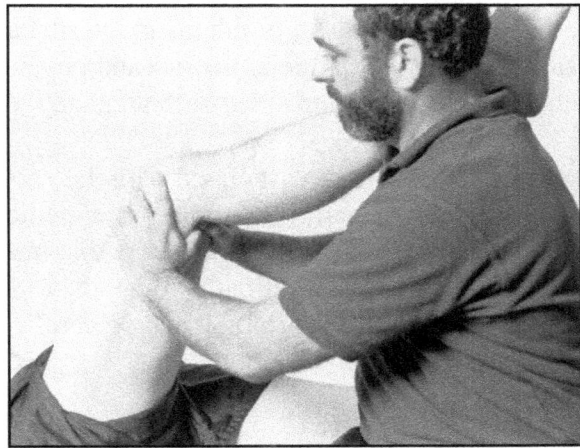

Popliteal Drainage Techniques

OSTEOPATHIC CLINICAL PROBLEM SOLVING

The osteopathic approach to patient care considers the patient as an integrated whole with dynamic interplay between structure and function. Problem solving begins with a detailed history and physical examination to consider all the possible etiologies related to the patient's present health status. From an osteopathic perspective, old illnesses and injuries leave their imprint on body structure and function, often making the patient more vulnerable to developing future problems. Even routine childbirth is considered to be a potential 'traumatic' event in the patient's history.

In the osteopathic approach to problem solving, patient complaints are evaluated independently, problem by problem, as well as in light of their relation to the patient's overall structure and function. This requires focused local inspection as well as examination of more distal structures for relevant clinical associations. Distal structures may have associations which can be primary (causal) or contributory to the area of the patient's chief complaint. Such associations can be mechanically linked (e.g. tendonitis), neurologically linked (e.g. radiculopathy), or viscerally linked (e.g. angina).

For example, a shoulder problem may be due to local injury to the capsule or to myotendinous insertions, or to more distal problems in the rib cage, thoracic outlet, cervical spine, gall-bladder, or opposite hip extensors. A good history and physical examination should serve to screen out these and other potential problems and help localize the clinical nature of the patient's chief complaint.

Management of problems associated with the patient's chief complaint may require emergent intervention or specialty referral for appropriate medical treatment as with an acute cholelithiasis or a stress fracture. In these situations, osteopathic manipulative treatment may also be helpful as adjunctive care. In many cases, osteopathic diagnosis and treatment alone will be effective in addressing the various mechanical, neurologic and visceral aspects and interelationships associated with the patient's chief complaint.

OSTEOPATHIC PROBLEM SOLVING MATRIX

An osteopathic screening examination with the goal of determining where the patient's problem areas are, should include: 1) gait analysis and 2) regional tests to evaluate structural landmarks, tissue resistance, and mobility. In addition to standard neurologic and orthopedic assessments, specific osteopathic tests should be carried out to evaluate possible nerve entrapment and myofascial/dural tension signs. Various approaches to locating areas of primary restrictions in the body and visceral structures can also be incorporated including palpating peripheral reflections of the cranial rhythmic impulse (CRI) or 'listening' techniques. Additionally, viscerosomatic or Chapman's reflexes may be present, also signifying the presence of visceral influences within the patient's musculoskeletal system.

Osteopathic scanning and segmental examinations further localize problems to specific areas and define their structural and functional characteristics so that specific therapeutic measures can be applied. Management of the whole patient requires consideration of the inter-relationships of the various problems identified, as well as further work-up of any potential health risks.

EXAMINATION OF THE ADULT PATIENT

SCREENING TESTS: To locate problems, regionally

1. Gait Analysis:

Forefoot pronation
Ankle eversion
Knee rotation and extension
Hip extension
Pelvic weight shift/mobility

Lumbar side bending
Thoracic cage mobility
Shoulder position
Arm swing
Head position

2. Static Landmarks

Scoliosis
Kyphosis
Lordosis

Head
Shoulder
Scapula
Iliac crest
Trochanter
Feet

3. Tissue Resistance to Pressure

4. Dynamic Testing

Standing
Pelvis
    Stork Test
Lumbar
    Rotation
    Side bending
    Flexion
Lower extremity
    Hip shift
    One leg stand
    Knee extension
Sitting
Upper extremity
    Forearm
    Pronation
Thoracic cage
    Side bending
    Rotation
    Flexion/extension
Cervical spine
    Side bending
    Rotation
    Flexion/extension

Supine
Pelvis
    Traction test
    Pelvic rock
Thoracolumbar spine
    Sit-up test
Head and cervical spine
    Head lift
    Jaw abduction
    Vault hold
Upper extremity
    Shoulder abduction
Lower Extremity
    Side bending
Costal cage
    Respiratory motion
    Sternal compliance
Prone
Pelvis
    Sacral rock
    Hip extension
Thoracic spine
    Push-up
Side-lying
Lower extremity
    Hip abduction

SCANNING TESTS: To localize segmentally, exact areas of dysfunction

1. Global "Listening"

2. Following Reflections of Peripheral CRI to Most Proximal Area of Assymetric Function

3. Tissue Texture Abnormalities

Moisture
Hardness

Temperature
Color

SEGMENTAL TESTING: To characterize dysfunction structurally and functionally

Ankle/foot
Knee
Hip/groin
Pelvis
Sacrum

Lumbar spine
Thoracic spine
Rib cage
Cervical spine
Head

Sternoclavicular
Acromioclavicular
Glenohumeral
Elbow
Wrist/hand

BIBLIOGRAPHY

Neuro Anatomic Relations

Burton H, Loewy AD, 1977, Projections to the spinal cord from the medullary somatosensory relay nuclei, J Comp Neurol, 173:773-792

Contreras RJ, Beckstead RM, Norgren R, 1982, The central projections of the trigeminal, facial, glossopharyngeal and vagus nerves: An autoradiographic study in the rat, J Autonomic Ner Sys, 6:303-322

Craig AD, 1978, Spinal and medullary input to the lateral cervical nucleus, J Comp Neurol, 181:729-744

Falls WM, Belt LA, Hruby RJ, 1997, Trigeminal efferent projections to sympathetic neurons in the rat...thoracic...spinal cord, AOA Research Conference 1997

Falls WM, Rice RE, Van Wagner JP, 1985, The dorsomedial portion trigeminal nucleus oralis (Vo) in the rat: Cytology and projections to the cerebellum, Somatosens Res, 3:89-118

Hayashi H., Sumino R, Sessle BJ, 1984, Functional organization of the trigeminal subnucleus interpolaris: Nociceptive and innocuous afferent inputs, projections to thalamus, cerebellum, and spinal cord, and descending modulation from periaqueductal gray, J Neurophysiol, 51:890-905

Matsushita M, Okado N, Ideda M, Hosoya LY, 1981, Descending projections from the spinal and mesencephalic nuclei of the trigeminal nerve to the spinal cord in the cat. A study with the horseradish perioxidase technique. J. Comp Neurol, 196:173-187

Millar J, 1979, Convergence of joint, cutaneous and muscle afferents onto cuneate neurons in the cat, Brain Research, 175:247-350

Peterson BW, Bilotto G. Goldberg J, Wilson VJ, 1981, Dynamics of vestibulo-ocular, vestibulo-collic, and cervicocollic reflexes, 1981, New York Academy of Sciences, pp 395-402

Rowe MJ, 1972, Responses of the trigeminal ganglion and brain stem neurons in the cat to mechanical and thermal stimulation of the face, Brain Res, 42:367-384

Ruggiero DA, Ross A., Reis DJ, 1981 Projections from the spinal trigeminal nucleus to the entire length of the spinal cord in the rat, Brain Res, 225:225-233

Sessle BJ, Greenwood LF, 1976, Inputs to trigeminal brain stem neurons from face, oral, tooth pulp and pharyngolaryngeal tissue, I. Responses to innocuous and noxious stimuli, Brain Res, 117:211-226

Neurosensory, Autonomic and Motor System Integration

Burgess PR, Perl ER, 1973, Cutaneous mechanoreceptors and nociceptors, in: Iggo A, ed, Handbook of Sensory Physiology, Vol 2: Somatosensory System, New York, Springer, pp 29-78

Coderre TJ, Katz J, Vaccarino AL, et al: Contribution of central neuroplasticity to pathological pain: Review of clinical and experimental evidence. Pain 52:259-285, 1993

Earl E. The dual sensory role of muscle spindles. *Phys Ther J.* 1965; 45:4.

Greenman PE (ed): Concepts and Mechanisms of Neuromuscular Functions. Springer-Verlag, Berlin, 1984

Hubbard DR, Berkoff GM: Myofascial trigger points show spontaneous needle EMG activity. *Spine.* 1993;18(13):1803-1807.

Janda V. Muscles, central nervous motor regulation and back problems. In: The neurobiologic mechanisms in manipulative therapy. Korr IM, ed. New York: Plenum Press, 1978; 27-41.

Kandel ER, Schwartz JH, Jessell TM, 1991, The Brain Stem and Reticular Core: Integration of Sensory and Motor Systems, in Kandel ER, Schwartz JH, Jessell TM, eds, Principles of Neural Science, Elsevier, New York, London, Amsterdam, pp 681-730

Korr IM. Sustained sympathicotonia as a factor in disease. In: The neurobiologic mechanisms of manipulative therapy. New York: Plenum Press, 1978; 229-268.

Manni E, Palmieri G, Marini KR, 1971, Extraocular muscle proprioception and the descending trigeminal nucleus, 33:195-204

Northrup GW: The Physiological Basis of Osteopathic Medicine. Postgraduate Institute of Osteopathic Medicine and Surgery, New York, 1970

Patterson MM: Louisa Burns Memorial Lecture, 1980: the spinal cord-active processor not passive transmitter. J Am osteopath Assoc 80:210, 1980

Patterson MM: Neurophysiologic system: integration and disintegration. p. 137. In Ward R (ed): Foundations for Osteopathic Medicine. Williams & Wilkins, Baltimore, 1997

Patterson MM: The Central Connection: Somatovisceral/Viscerosomatic Interaction. American Academy of osteopathy, Indianapolis, 1992

Sato, A, 1989, Reflex modulation of visceral functions by somatic afferent activity, in: Patterson NM, Howell JN, eds, The Central Connection: Somatovisceral/Viscerosomatic Interaction, 1989 International Symposium, American Academy of Osteopathy, Indianapolis, pp 53-72

Schaible HG, Neugebauer V, Cervero F, Schmidt RF, 1991, Changes in tonic descending inhibition of spinal neurons with articular input during the development of acute arthritis in the cat.

Schmidt RF, 1973, Control of the access of afferent activity to somatosensory pathways, in: Iggo, ed, Somatosensory System, Handbook of Sensory Physiology, Vol 2, Springer, Heidelberg

VanBuskirk RL, 1990, Nociceptive reflexes and the somatic dysfunction: A Model, JAOA, 90:9:792-809

Willard FH: Autonomic nervous system. p. 53. In Ward R (ed): Foundations for Osteopathic Medicine. Williams & Wilkins, Baltimore, 1997

Wilson VJ, 1988, The tonic neck reflex: spinal circuitry, in, Peterson B,Richmond F; eds, Control of head movement, Oxford University Press, New York, Oxford, pp

Wilson, VJ. Inhibition in the central nervous system. *Sci Am.* 1966;5:102-108.

Zhu Y, Halderman S, Starr A, Seffinger MA, Su-Hwan S, 1993, Paraspinal Muscle evoked cerebral potentials in patients with unilateral back pain, Spine, 18:8:1096-1101

Chemical and Mechanical Properties of Musculoskeletal System and Their Relation to Connective Tissues

Abitbol, MM, Energy Storage in the Vertebral Columns. In: Second Interdisciplinary World Congress on Low Back Pain. The Integrated Function of the Lumbar Spine and Sacroiliac Joints. Vleeming A, Mooney V, Snijders C, Dorman T. (eds). San Diego, Nov 9-11, 1995, p. 257.

Adams MA, Dolan P, Hutton WC (1988). The lumbar spine in backward bending. Spine 13 9 1019-26.

Adams MA, Hutton WC (1980). The effect of posture on the role of the apophyseal joints in resisting intervertebral compressive force. J Bone Jt Surg 62-B 358-362.

Adams MA, McNally DM, Chinn H, Dolan P (1994). Posture and the compressive strength of the lumbar spine. International Society of Biomechanics Award Paper. Clin Biomech 9 5-14.

Adams, MA, Posture and Spinal Mechanisms During Lifting. In: Second Interdisciplinary World Congress on Low Back Pain. The Integrated Function of the Lumbar Spine and Sacroiliac Joints. Vleeming A, Mooney V, Snijders C, Dorman T. (eds). San Diego, Nov 9-11, 1995, p. 17.

Ahmed M, Bjurholm A, Kreicbergs A, Schultzberg M: Neuropeptide Y, tyrosine hydroxylase and vasoactive intestinal polypeptide-immunoreactive nerve fibers in the vertebral bodies, disc, dura mater, and spinal ligaments of the rat lumbar spine. Spine 18: 268-273, 1993.

Alexander, R.McN & Bennet-Clark, H.C. (1977) Storage of elastic strain energy in muscle and other tissues. Nature 265 : 114-117.

Alexander, R.McN., Dimery, N.J. & Ker, R.F. (1995) Elastic structures in the back and their role in galloping in some mammals. J. Zool., Lond. (A) 207 : 467-482.

Alexander, R-McN., Elasticity in Mammalian Backs. In: Second Interdisciplinary World Congress on Low Back Pain. The Integrated Function of the Lumbar Spine and Sacroiliac Joints. Vleeming A, Mooney V, Snijders C, Dorman T. (eds). San Diego, Nov 9-11, 1995, p. 7.

Aspden RM, Bornstein NH, Hukins DWL: Collagen organization in the interspinous ligament and its relationship to tissue function. J Anatomy 155: 141-151, 1987.

Basbaum AI, Levine JD: The contributions of the nervous system to inflammation and inflammatory disease. Can J. Physiol. Pharmacol. 69: 647-651, 1991.

Bennett, M.B., Ker, R.F. & Alexander, R.McN. (1987) Elastic properties of structures in the tails of cetaceans (Phocaena and Lagenorhynchus) and their effect on the energy cost of swimming. J. Zool. Lond. 211 : 177-192.

Blickhan, R. & Cheng, J.-Y. (1994) Energy storage by elastic mechanisms in the tail of large swimmers - a re-evaluation. J. Theor. Biol. 168 : 315-336.

Bogduk N, Macintosh JE, Pearcy MJ (1992). A universal model of the lumbar back muscles in the upright position. Spine 17 8 897-913.

Crisco JJ, Panjabi MM: The intersegmental and multisegmental muscles of the lumbar spine: a biomechanical model comparing lateral stabilizing potential. Spine 16: 793-799, 1991.

Dolan P, Adams MA, Hutton WC (1988). Commonly adopted postures and their effect on the lumbar spine. Spine 13 197-201.

Dolan P, Earley M, Adams MA (1994). Bending and compressive stresses acting on the lumbar spine during lifting activities. J Biomech 27 1237-1248.

Dolan P, Mannion AF, Adams MA (1994). Passive tissues help the back muscles to generate extensor moments during lifting. J Biomech 27 1077-1085.

Dorman, T. (1992) Storage and release of elastic energy in the pelvis: dysfunction, diagnosis and treatment. J. orthopaed. Med. 14 : 54-62.

Dunn, MG, Silver FH. Viscoelastic behavior of human connective tissues: relative contribution of viscous and elastic components. Connect Tissue Res 1983;12

Floyd WF, Silver PHS (1955). The functions of the erectores spinae muscles in certain movements and postures in man. J. Physiol. 129 184-203.

Gál, J.M. (1992) Spinal flexion and locomotor energetics in kangaroo, monkey, and tiger. Can J. Zool. 70 : 2444-2451.

Gál, J.M. (1993a) Mammalian spinal biomechanics. I. Static and dynamic mechanical properties of intact intervertebral joints. J. exp. Biol. 174 : 247-280.

Gál, J.M. (1993b) Mammalian spinal biomechanics. II. Intevertebral lesion experiments and mechanisms of bending resistance. J. exp. Biol. 174 : 281-297.

Gracovetsky, S, Farfan HF, Lamy C. The mechanism of the lumbar spine. Spine 6:249-262, 1981.

Gracovetsky, SA. Locomotion. Linking the Spinal Engine with the Legs. In: Second Interdisciplinary World Congress on Low Back Pain. The Integrated Function of the Lumbar Spine and Sacroiliac Joints. Vleeming A, Mooney V, Snijders C, Dorman T. (eds). San Diego, Nov 9-11, 1995, p. 169.

Hoyt, D.F. & Taylor, C.R. (1981) Gaits and the energetics of locomotion in horses. Nature 292 : 239-240.

Hubbard RP, Mechanical Behavior of Connective Tissue. In Concepts and Mechanisms of Neuromuscular Functions (ed) PE Greenman Springer Neulog 1984; 47-54.

Jonsson Jr H, et al, Findings and outcome in whiplash-type neck distortions, Spine, 19:2733-2743, 1994.

Katake K (1961). Studies on the strength of human skeletal muscles. J Kyoto Pref Med Univ 69 463-483.

Ker, R.F., Bennett, M.B., Bibby, S.R., Kester, R.C. & Alexander, R.McN. (1987) The spring in the arch of the human foot. Nature 325 : 147-149.

Levine J, Collier DH, Basbaum AI, Moskowitz MA, Helms CA: Hypothesis: the nervous system may contribute to the pathophysiology of rheumatoid artritis. J. Rheumatol. 12: 406-411, 1985.

Macintosh J, Bogduk N: The biomechanics of the lumbar multifidus. Clin. Biomech. 1: 205-213, 1986.

MacIntosh JE, Bogduk N, Pearcy MJ (1993). The effects of flexion on the geometry and actions of the lumbar erector spinae. Spine 18 884-93.

McGill SM, Patt N, Norman RW (1988). Measurement of the trunk musculature of active males using CT scan radiography: implications for force and moment generating capacity about the L4/L5 joint. J Biomech 21 4 329-41.

Mense, Siegfried, Pathophysiologic Basis of Muscle Pain Syndromes. 1997 PM & R Clinics 8:1;23-53.

Myklebust JB, Pintar F, Yoganandan N, Cusick JF et al (1988). Tensile strength of spinal ligaments. Spine 13 526-531.

Page LE. The role of fasciae in the maintenance of structural integrity. Newark, OH: American Academy of Osteopathy Yearbook, 1952; 70-73.

Panjabi MM, White AA. In White, AA, Panjabi,MM (eds): Clinical Biomechanics of the Spine. Philadelphia, J.B. Lippincott Company, 1990.

Portanova R: Endocrine system and body unity: osteopathic principles at a chemical level. p. 83. In Ward R (ed): Foundations for Osteopathic Medicine. Williams & Wilkins, Baltimore, 1997.

Potvin JR, Norman RW, McGill SM (1991). Reduction in anterior shear forces on the L4/L5 disc by the lumbar musculature. Clin Biomech 6 88-96.

Pursloe PP (1989). Strain-induced reorientation of an intramuscular connective tissue network: implications for passive muscle elasticity. J Biomech 22 21-31.

Selye, H: The stress of life. Mc-Graw Hill Book Co., New York, 1956.

Smeathers, J.E. & Joanes, D.N. (1988) Dynamic compression properties of human intervertebral joints: a comparison between fresh and thawed specimens. J. Biomechan. 21 : 425-433.

Snijders CJ, Vleeming A, Stoeckart R: Transfer of lumbosacral load to iliac bones and legs. Part I: Biomechanics of self-bracing of the sacroiliac joints and its significance for treatment and exercise. Clin. Biomech. 8: 285-294, 1993a.

Snijders, CJ, Biomechanics of Sacroiliac Joint Stability; Validation Experiments on the Concept of Self-Locking. In: Second Interdisciplinary World Congress on Low Back Pain. The Integrated Function of the Lumbar Spine and Sacroiliac Joints. Vleeming A, Mooney V, Snijders C, Dorman T. (eds). San Diego, Nov 9-11, 1995, p. 75.

Taylor RB, Bioenergetics of Man, AAO Yearbook. 1958: 91-96.

Viidik A, Adaptability of connective tissue. In: Biochemistry of exercise VI. Saltin B, ed. Champaign: Human Kinetics Publishers, 1986; 545-562.

Viidik A. Interdependence between structure and function in collagenous tissues. In: Biology of collagen. Viidik A, Vuust J, (eds) New York: Academic Press, Harcourt, Brace, Jovanovich, 1985; 2 56-562.

Vleeming A, et al. Relations between form and function in the sacroiliac joint: Part II: biomechanical aspects. Spine 1990; 15:133-136.

Vleeming A, Stoeckart R, Snijders CJ: The sacrotuberous ligament: a conceptual approach to its dynamic role in stabilizing the sacroiliac joint. Clin. Biomech. 4: 201-203, 1989a.

Vleeming A, Van Wingerdan JP, Snijders CJ, Stoeckart R, Stijnen T: Load application to the sacrotuberous ligament; influences on sacroiliac joint mechanics. Clin. Biomech. 4: 204-209, 1989b.

Willard FH: Neuroendocrine, immune system, and homeostatis. p. 107. In Ward R (ed): Foundations for Osteopathic Medicine. Williams & Wilkins, Baltimore, 1997.

Willard FH: Nociception and the neuroendocrine immune connection. In Proceedings of the 1991 American Academy of Osteopathy International Symposium. University Classics Ltd, Athens, OH, 1991.

Yamashita T, Cavanaugh JM, El-Bohy AA, Getchell TV, King Al Mechanosensitive afferent units in the lumbar facet joint. J Bone Joint Surg (Am) 72-A: 865-870, 1990.

Functional Anatomy of Myofascial and Fascial-ligamentous Tissues

Alaranta H, Tallroth K, Soukla A, Heliovaara M (1993): Fat content of lumbar extensor muscles and low back disability: A radiographic and clinical comparison. *Journal of Spinal Disorders* 6(2): 137-140.

Bagnall KM, et al. The histochemical composition of vertebral muscle. Spine 1984; 9:470-473.

Bagnall KM, Ford DM, McFadden KD, Greenhill BJ and Raso VJ (1984): The histochemical composition of human vertebral muscle. *Spine* 9: 470-473.

Becker RF. The meaning of fascia and fascial continuity. *Osteopath Am.* 1975;3:8-32.

Bogduk, N, Twomey LT: Clinical Anatomy of the Lumbar Spine. 2nd edition. Melbourne, Churchill Livingstone, 1991.

Bogduk, N: A reappraisal of the anatomy of the human lumbar erector spinae. J. Anat. 131: 525-540, 1980.

Bogduk, N: The Applied Anatomy of the Thoracolumbar Fascia. Spine 1984; 9:2, 169-170.

Cathie, A.G. American Academy of Osteopathy Year Book 1977. Fascia of the body in relation to function and manipulative therapy. 1974:81.

Cathie, A.G. American Academy of Osteopathy Year Book 1977. Fascia, considerations of, and its relation to disease of the musculoskeletal system. 1974:85.

Cooper RG, Clair Forbes WST, Jayson MIV (1992): Radiographic demonstration of paraspinal muscle wasting in patients with chronic low back pain. *British Journal of Rheumatology* 31: 389-394.

Dananberg, HJ, The action of Lower Extremity and its Relationship to Lumbo-Sacral Function. In: Second Interdisciplinary World Congress on Low Back Pain: The Integrated Function of the Lumbar Spine and Sacroiliac Joints. San Diego, November 9-11, 1995, p. 461.

Erlingheuser, R.F.: The circulation of the cerebrospinal fluid through the connective tissue system. In Academy of Applied Osteopathy year book 1959.

Hanson P, Sonesson B: The anatomy of the iliolumbar ligament. Arch Phys Med Rehabil 75: 1245-1246, 1994.

Heylings DJA: Supraspinous and interspinous ligaments of the human lumbar spine. J. Anat. 125: 127-131, 1978.

Hukins DWL, Kirby MC, Sikoryn TA, Aspden RM, Cox AJ: Comparison of structure, mechanical properties, and function of lumbar spinal ligaments. Spine 15: 787-795.

Korkala O, Gronblad M, et al., Immunohistochemical Demonstration of Nociceptors in the Ligamentous Structure of the Lumbar Spine. Spine, Vol. 10, No. 2, Mar. 85, pp 156-157.

Korkala O, Gronblad M, Liesi P, Karaharju E: Immunohistochemical demonstration of nociceptors in the ligamentous structures of the lumbar spine. Spine 10: 156-157, 1985.

Luk KDK, Ho HC, Leong JCY: The iliolumbar ligament a study of its anatomy development and clinical significance. J. Bone Joint Surg. 68B: 197-200, 1986.

Page, L. E.: The role of the fasciae in the maintenance of structural integrity. In Academy of Applied Osteopathy year book 1952, p. 70.

Ramsey RH: The anatomy of the ligamenta flava. Clin. Orthped. Rel. Res. 44: 129-140, 1966.

Sapega, AA. Biophysical Factors in Range-of-Motion Exercise. In: The Physician and Sports Medicine, Vol. 9, No. 12, December 1981.

Snyder, G.E.: Embryology and physiology of fascia. J. Osteopath Cranial Ass., pp. 4-15, 1954.

Snyder, G.E.: Fasciae - Applied anatomy and physiology. In Academy of Applied Osteopathy year book 1956, p. 66.

Taylor JR and Twomey LT (1993): Acute injuries to cervical joints: an autopsy study of neck sprain. *Spine* 18:9:1115-1122.

Tesh KM, Shaw Dunn J, Evans JH (1987). The abdominal muscles and vertebral stability. Spine 12 501-508.

Tracy MF, Gibson MJ, Szpryt EP, Rutherford A, Corlett EN (1989). The geometry of the muscles of the lumbar spine determined by magnetic resonance imaging. Spine 14 186-193.

Tveit P, Daggfeldt K, Hetland S, Thorstensson A (1994). Erector spinae lever arm length variations with changes in spinal curvature. Spine 19 2 199-204.

Uitto J, and Perejda AJ. Structure and biology of the components of the extracellular matrix. In: Connective tissue diseases: the molecular pathology of the extracellular matrix. New York: Marcel Dekker; 1987; 12-3-100.

van Wingerden, JP, Interaction of Spine and Legs: Influence of Hamstring Tension on Lumbo-Pelvic Rhythm. In: Second Interdisciplinary World Congress on Low Back Pain: The Integrated Function of the Lumbar Spine and Sacroiliac Joints. San Diego, November 9-11, 1995, p. 109.

Vleeming A, et al. Relation between form and function in the sacroiliac joint: Part I: clinical anatomical aspects. Spine 1990; 15:130-132.

Vleeming A, Pool-Goudzwaard AL, Stoeckart R, van Wingerden J-P, Snijders CJ (1995). The posterior layer of the thoracolumbar fascia. Its function in load transfer from spine to legs. Spine 20 753-8.

Willard FH, The Lumbosacral Connection: The Ligamentous Structure of the Low Back and its Relation to Back Pain. In: Second Interdisciplinary World Congress on Low Back Pain: The Integrated Function of the Lumbar Spine and Sacroiliac Joints. San Diego, November 9-11, 1995, p. 29.

Woo S-L, An K-N, Arnoczky SP, Wayne JS, Fithian DC, Myers DS. Anatomy, biology, and biomechanics of tendon, ligament, and rotation. In: Simon SR, ed. *Orthopedic Basic Science*. American Academy of Orthopedic Surgeons; 1994-45-88.

Yahia L-H, Garzon S, Strykowski H, Rivard C-H: Ultrastructure of the human interspinous ligament and ligamentum flavum: a preliminary study. Spine 15: 262-268, 1990.

Yamamoto I, Panjabi MM, Oxland TR, Crisco JJ: The role of the iliolumbar ligament in the lumbosacral junction. Spine 15: 1138-1141, 1990.

Principles of Diagnosis, Treatment and Problem Solving

Becker RE. Diagnostic touch - its principles and application. In: Barnes M.W., ed. *Academy of Applied Osteopathy Yearbooks*. Indianapolis, Ind: American Academy of Osteopathy; Part I. 1963:32-40. Parts II and III. 1964:153-166. Part IV. 1965:165-177.

Bookhout MR: Exercise in somatic dysfunction. Phys Med Rehabil Clin North Am 7:845, 1996.

Cantu RL: Myofascial Manipulation: Theory and Clinical Application. Aspen, Gaithersburg, MD, 1992.

Chila A 1997, Fascial-Ligamentous Release, Indirect Approach, in, RC Ward, ed, Foundations for Osteopathic Medicine, Williams and Wilkins, Baltimore, p 819-830.

Greenman PE, 1995, Principles of Manual Medicine, 2nd ed. Williams and Wilkins, Baltimore.

Janda V: Treatment of chronic back pain. J. Manual Med 6: 166, 1992.

Lippincott HA: The osteopathic technique of Wm. G. Sutherland, D.O. In Academy of Applied Osteopathy year book 1949.

Lippincott HA: Respiratory technic according to the principles of Wm. G. Sutherland, D.O. In Academy of Applied Osteopathy year book 1948.

Little KE, Toward More Effective Manipulative Management of chronic myofascial strain and stress syndromes. Journal of ADA 1969: 68:675-685.

Simons DG, Travell JG. Low back pain, Part 2: torso muscles. *Post Grad Med.* 1983;73(2):81-92.

Still A.T.: The philosophy and mechanical principles of osteopathy. Hudson-Kimberly Publishing Co., Kansas City, Mo., 1902, p. 60.

Travell JG, Simons DG. *Myofascial Pain and Dysfunction: The Trigger Point Manual: The Upper Extremities.* Vol. I. Baltimore, Md: Williams & Wilkins; 1983.

Travell JG, Simons DG. *Myofascial Pain and Dysfunction: The Trigger Point Manual: The Lower Extremities.* Vol. II. Baltimore, Md: Williams & Wilkins; 1992:547.

Ward R (ed): Foundations for Osteopathic Medicine. Williams & Wilkins, Baltimore, 1997.

Ward R, Myofascial Release Concepts in Rational Manual Therapies. (eds) Basmajian & Nyberg. Williams & Wilkins 1993.

Ward R: Glossary of osteopathic terminology. J. Am Osteopath Assoc 80; 552, 1981.

Ward RC, 1997, Integrated Neuromusculoskeletal and Myofascial Release, in, RC Ward, ed, Foundations for Osteopathic Medicine, Williams and Wilkins, Baltimore, p 844-850.

Ward RC, 1997, Integrated Neuromusculoskeletal Techniques for Specific Areas, ibid, Chapter 63, in, RC Ward, ed, Foundations for Osteopathic Medicine, Williams and Wilkins, Baltimore, p 851-900.

Clinical Importance of Fascia and Fascial Relations

Arena JG, Sherman RA, Bruno GM, et al: Electgromyographic recordings of 5 types of low back pain subjects and non-pain controls in different positions. *Pain* 1989;37:57-65.

Beal MC: The sacroiliac problem: review of anatomy, mechanics, and diagnosis. JAOA 81: 667-679, 1982.

Bennett RM. Myofascial pain syndromes and the fibromyalgia syndrome: a comparative analysis. *J. Man Med.* 1991;6(1):34-45.

Bilkey W: Involvement of fascia in mechanical pain syndromes. J Manual Med 6:157, 1992.

Cathie AG, England RW, eds. The clinical importance of fascia. Newark, OH: Academy of Applied Osteopathy Yearbook, 1968; 87-103.

Cathie, AG. The fascia of the body in relation to function and manipulative therapy. In: *The American Academy of Osteopathy Yearbook.* Indianapolis, Ind: American Academy of Osteopathy; 1974:81-87.

Cooper GJ. Clinical considerations on fascia in diagnosis and treatment. Newark, OH: American Academy of Osteopathy Yearbook, 1977; 73-84.

Dorman T.A.: Energy Efficiency during Human Walking Before and After Prolotherapy. In: Second Interdisciplinary World Congress on Low Back Pain: The Integrated Function of the Lumbar Spine and Sacroiliac Joints. San Diego, November 9-11, 1995, p. 637.

Dorman T.A.: Failure of Self Bracing at the Sacroiliac Joints: The Slipping Clutch Syndrome. In: Second Interdisciplinary World Congress on Low Back Pain: The Integrated Function of the Lumbar Spine and Sacroiliac Joints. San Diego, November 9-11, 1995, p. 651.

Ellestad SM, Nagle RV, Boesler DR, et al: Electromyographic and skin resistance responses to osteopathic manipulative treatment for low-back pain. JAOA 1988;88:991-997.

Hench PK. Myofascial pain syndromes and clinical insights into musculoskeletal problems. *Myology*. 1980;5(1):5.

Hoyt WH, Hunt HH, Jr, DePauw MA, et al: Electromyographic assessment of chronic low-back pain syndrome. JAOA 1981;80:728-730.

Hult L, The Munkfors Investigation: A study of the frequency and causes of the still neck-brachialgia and lumbago-sciatica syndromes, as well as observations on certain signs and symptoms from the dorsal spine and the joints of the extremities in industrial and forest workers. *Acta Orthop Scand* 1954; (suppl 16):5-76.

Jaeger B, Reeves JL: Quantification of changes in myofascial trigger point sensitivity with pressure algometer following passive stretch. *Pain* 27:203-210, 1986.

Kauffman, C.H.: Connective tissue and osteopathy (Resume by A. R. Becker). In Academy of Applied Osteopathy year book 1945.

Kuslich SD, Ulstrom CL, Michael CJ (1991). The tissue origin of low back pain and sciatica. Orthop Clin N Amer 22 2 181-7.

Lee D: Instability of the Sacroiliac Joint and the Consequences to Gait. In: Second Interdisciplinary World Congress on Low Back Pain: The Integrated Function of the Lumbar Spine and Sacroiliac Joints. San Diego, November 9-11, 1995, p. 471.

Magoun, H.I.: Fascia in the writings of A. T. Still. *J. Osteopath Cranial Ass.* pp. 16-25 1954.

Mense S: Nociception from skeletal muscle in relation to clinical muscle pain. *Pain* 54:241-289, 1993.

Pearcy, M., Portek, I., & Shephere, J., The Effect of Low-Back Pain on Lumbar Spinal Movements Measured by Three Dimensional X-ray Analysis, *Spine*, Vol. 10, No. 2, Mar. 85, pp. 150-153.

Peterson B: Postural Balance and Imbalance. American Academy of Osteopathy, Indianapolis, 1983.

Rolf, I.P.: Postural release, an exploration in structural dynamics. Published by the author. New York, 1957, p. 3.

Roy SH, DeLuca CJ, Casavant DA (1989): Lumbar muscle fatigue and chronic low back pain. *Spine* 14: 992-1001.

Sherman RA: Relationships between strength of low back muscle contraction and reported intensity of chronic low back pain. *Am J Phys Med* 1985;64:190-200.

Sihvonen T, Partanen J., Hanninen O, Soimakallio S (1991): Electric behaviour of low back muscles during lumbar pelvic rhythm in low back pain patients and healthy controls. *Archives of Physical Medicine and Rehabilitation* 72: 1080-1087.

Simons DG. Muscle pain syndromes. *J Man Med.* 1991;6:18.

Strait B, Kuchera ML. Osteopathic manipulation for patients with confirmed mild, modest, and moderate carpal tunnel syndrome. *JAOA.* 1994;94(8):673.

Sucher BM. Thoracic outlet syndrome-a myofascial variant: Part 1. Pathology and diagnosis. J Am Osteopath Assoc 1990; 90(8):686-704.

Sucher BM. Thoracic outlet syndrome-a myofascial variant: Part 2. Treatment. J Am Osteopath Assoc 1990; 90(9):810-823.

Sucher BM. Thoracic outlet syndrome-a myofascial variant: Part 3. Structural and postural considerations J Am Osteopath Assoc 1993; 93(3):

Travell J, Rinzler SH. The myofasical genesis of pain. Postgrad Med 1952; 11:425-34.

Twomey LT, Taylor JR, Oliver MJ. Sustained flexion loading, rapid extension loading of the lumbar spine, and the physical therapy of related injuries. 1988. Physiotherapy Practice, 4:129-138.

Vleeming A: Low back pain: the integrated function of the lumbar spine and sacroiliac joints. In Proceedings of the 2nd Interdisciplinary World Congress, San Diego, 1995.

Vleeming A: Movement, the Pelvis, and Low Back Pain: An Interdisciplinary Approach. Churchill Livingstone, Edinburgh, 1999.

Course Schedule
Level I- Day 1

8:00 am	*(9:00 am)*		Course Introduction/ Announcements
8:45 am	*(9:45 am)*		Myofascial Release Concept •Basic Concepts and Terminology
9:45 am	*(10:45 am)*		Break
10:15 am	*(11:15 am)*		Myofascial Release Concept •Principles of Treatment •Demonstration
11:45 am	*(12:45 am)*		Lunch
1:00 pm	*(2:00 pm)*		Point of Entry: Thorax/ Costal Cage Demonstration and Treatment •Thoracolumbar junction- prone (direct stretch) •Lower costal cage- supine and seated (indirect) •Upper thorax- supine (indirect, direct stretch x2)
2:45 pm	*(3:45 pm)*		Break
3:15 pm	*(4:15 pm)*		Point of Entry: Lower Extremity Demonstration and Treatment •Ankle- supine (indirect) •Knee- supine (direct stretch) •Single lower extremity- supine (direct unwinding)
5:00 pm	*(6:00 pm)*		Adjourn

Course Schedule
Level I- Day 2

8:00   am   (*9:00 am*)   Review and Questions

8:30   am   (*9:30 am*)   Point of Entry: Thorax/ Costal Cage
                               Demonstration and Treatment
                               •Scapulothoracic Release- side-lying (indirect, direct unwinding)
                               •Upper costal cage- supine and seated (direct pumping, direct
                               unwinding)

9:45   am   (*10:45 am*)   Break

10:15 am   (*11:15 am*)   Point of Entry: Upper Extremity
                               Demonstration and Treatment
                               •Finger- seated (indirect)
                               •Single and double upper extremity- supine (direct unwinding)

11:45 am   (*12:45 am*)   Lunch

1:00   pm   (*2:00 pm*)   Point of Entry: Cervical Spine
                               Demonstration and Treatment
                               •Cervicothoracic twist- supine (direct stretch)
                               •Lateral cervical spine - supine (direct unwinding)
                               •Thoracic outlet- seated (indirect)

2:45   pm   (*3:45 pm*)   Break

3:15   pm   (*4:15 pm*)   Point of Entry: Lumbosacral Spine and Pelvis
                               Demonstration and Treatment
                               •Lumbosacral spine- prone (direct unwinding, direct pumping,
                               direct stretch)
                               •Pelvis- prone (direct stretch, direct pumping, indirect
                               unwinding)
                               •Pelvis- supine (direct stretch, direct pumping)
                               •Pubis- supine (direct stretch)

5:00   pm   (*6:00 pm*)   Adjourn

Course Schedule
Level I- Day 3

8:00 am	(*9:00 am*)	Review and Questions
8:30 am	(*9:30 am*)	Point of Entry: Sacrum

Demonstration and Treatment
- Abdomen/ visceral release- supine (indirect)
- Sternum- supine (direct unwinding)

9:45 am	(*10:45 am*)	Break
10:15 am	(*11:15 am*)	Discussion- open time
11:45 am	(*12:45 am*)	Lunch
1:00 pm	(*2:00 pm*)	Two Operator Technique

- Sacrum and double upper extremity (direct unwinding)
- Upper thorax and double lower extremity- supine (direct unwinding)

2:45 pm	(*3:45 pm*)	Break
3:15 pm	(*4:15 pm*)	Multiple Operator Technique

- Four operator technique- supine (indirect)

4:45 pm	(*5:45 pm*)	Closing
5:00 pm	(*6:00 pm*)	Adjourn

Course Schedule
Level II-Day 1

8:00 am   *(9:00 am)*   Lecture - Review of physiology of connective tissue

                                        •Review of myofascial release concept

8:45 am   *(9:45 am)*   *Table Session* - Myofascial screening examination

9:30 am   *(10:30 am)*   Break

9:45 am   *(10:45 am)*   Release enhancing maneuvers

10:00 am   *(11:00 am)*   *Table Session* - Review techniques from Myofascial Release, Level I

                                        •Demonstration and practice

11:45 am   *(12:45 pm)*   Lunch

1:00 pm   *(2:00 pm)*   Lecture- Cranial nerve facilitation in it's relation to central and peripheral pain mechanisms and proprioceptive function

                                        •Anatomic considerations

                                        •Influence of traumatic mechanical forces

1:20 pm   *(2:20 pm)*   Assessment and treatment protocols utilizing cranial nerve and proprioceptive facilitation maneuvers

2:45 pm   *(3:45 pm)*   Break

3:00 pm   *(4:00 pm)*   *Table Session* - Assessment and treatment protocols utilizing cranial nerve and proprioceptive facilitation maneuvers

5:00 pm   *(6:00 pm)*   Adjourn

Course Schedule
Level II-Day 2

8:00 am	(*9:00 am*)	Lecture- Use of fulcrum points to facilitate diagnostic touch and therapeutic potency
8:30 am	(*9:30 am*)	*Table Session* - Fulcrum point treatment sequence for the lower half of the body
10:00 am	(*11:00 am*)	Break
10:20 am	(*11:20 am*)	*Table Session* - Fulcrum point treatment sequence for the upper half of the body
11:45 am	(*12:45 pm*)	Lunch
1:00 pm	(*2:00 pm*)	Lecture - Craniofascial continuity and the core envelope
1:30 pm	(*2:30 pm*)	*Table Session* - Core envelope release

- Brachial sheath

- Sciatic sheath

2:45 pm	(*3:45 pm*)	Break
3:00 pm	(*4:00 pm*)	*Table Session* - Dynamic extremity release

- Upper extremity patterning/sequencing - side-lying

5:00 pm	(*6:00 pm*)	Adjourn

Course Schedule
Level II-Day 3

8:00 am   (*9:00 am*)   Questions; Discussion

8:30 am   (*9:30 am*)   *Table Session* - Dynamic extremity release

                                        •Lower extremity patterning/sequencing - supine

9:45 am   (*10:45 am*)   Break

10:00 am   (*11:00 am*)   Osteopathic technique of William G. Sutherland, DO

10:30 am   (*11:30 am*)   *Table Session* - Osseous techniques

11:45 am   (*12:45 pm*)   Lunch

1:00 pm   (*2:00 pm*)   *Table Session* - Non-osseous techniques

3:00 pm   (*4:00 pm*)   Adjourn

SFIMMS SERIES IN NEUROMUSCULOSKELETAL MEDICINE

AUTHORS: Harry Friedman D.O., Wolfgang Gilliar D.O., Jerel Glassman D.O.

Osteopathic approaches to patient care offer the practitioner a variety of problem-solving and treatment options. Palpatory skill development establishes a basis for diagnostic assessment of neuromusculoskeletal function and its integrative role in maintaining health and overcoming disease. Osteopathic treatment and problem-solving skills apply a holistic approach that considers the therapeutic response of the whole patient. A variety of diagnostic and treatment methods have been developed to maximize outcomes.

This series of Osteopathic manipulative medicine texts presents a comprehensive course of instruction, including theory, palpation, diagnosis, and treatment. The thoughtful student will appreciate the detail and clarity of topic presentation and the sequence of skills development. Quality close-up photographic visuals accurately depict the table sessions using human and anatomic models.

COUNTERSTRAIN APPROACHES IN OSTEOPATHIC MANIPULATIVE MEDICINE

* Basic and intermediate level instructional manual
* Theoretical principles of indirect technique and spontaneous release by positioning
* Diagnostic application of tender point palpation for each body region
* Multiple therapeutic procedures presented for each tender point

MYOFASCIAL AND FASCIAL-LIGAMENTOUS APPROACHES IN OSTEOPATHIC MANIPULATIVE MEDICINE

* Basic and advanced level instructional manual
* Detailed connective tissue anatomy and physiology
* Theoretical principles of myofascial and fascial-ligamentous release
* Diagnostic and treatment approaches for each body region, including a myofascial screening exam
* Release enhancing maneuvers and multiple operator techniques
* Includes approaches of Dr.'s Ward, Chila, Becker, Barral and Sutherland

OSTEOPATHIC MANIPULATIVE MEDICINE APPROACHES TO THE PRIMARY RESPIRATORY MECHANISM

* Basic, intermediate, and advanced level instructional manual
* Anatomic relations and physiologic principles underlying the cranial concept
* Palpation exercises designed to facilitate diagnostic touch throughout the body
* Diagnostic and treatment approaches focus on fluid, membranous (dural), muscular, articular and bony aspects of the cranial mechanism, including a cranial screening exam
* Includes multiple operator techniques and approaches to infants and children

FUNCTIONAL METHODS IN OSTEOPATHIC MANIPULATIVE MEDICINE

* Presents Functional Methods approach developed by William L Johnston DO FAAO
* 2 basic level courses to cover all body regions
* Presents a unique palpation based understanding of the functional relationships between all body regions
* Diagnostic principles based on passive motion testing
* Treatment elegantly applies palpation based findings to restore proper relationships between body regions

email: admin@sfimms.com
www.sfimms.com